T0304689

Pragmatic Healthcare Ethnography

This practical and accessible textbook provides an overview of the key principles for conducting ethnography in healthcare settings. Shedding new light on healthcare delivery and experiences, ethnographic research methods provide a useful set of tools for observing how people act in the world and help us understand why people act as they do. Increasingly recognized for their explanatory power, especially around behavior and social context, ethnographic methods are an invaluable approach for understanding challenges and processes in healthcare services and delivery.

This guide takes the reader step-by-step through the research process, from grant writing and study design to data collection and analysis. Each chapter, illustrated by a range of examples, introduces ethnographic concepts and techniques, considers how to apply them in pragmatic research, and includes suggestions for tips and tricks. An in-depth case study describing real-world ethnographic research in a healthcare setting follows each chapter to demonstrate both the "how to" and the value of ethnographic approaches. The case studies discuss why the researcher used ethnography, the specific approach taken, the setting for the work, and key lessons that demonstrate ethnographic principles covered in the related chapter.

This is an essential text for researchers from a range of health-related backgrounds new to ethnographic methods, including students taking courses on qualitative research methods in health, implementation science, and applied anthropology.

Alison B. Hamilton is a VA Research Career Scientist and Implementation Research Director with the Center for the Study of Healthcare Innovation, Implementation, and Policy at the VA Greater Los Angeles Healthcare System, a Professor-in-Residence in the University of California Los Angeles (UCLA) Department of Psychiatry and Biobehavioral Science, David Geffen School of Medicine, and an Honorary Professor in the Department of Psychiatry and Mental Health, University of Cape Town, South Africa. Her research interests include gender and health, mental health, implementation science, and research methods.

Gemmae M. Fix is an Associate Professor at Boston University Chobanian & Avedisian School of Medicine and a Research Health Scientist with the Center for Healthcare Organization and Implementation Research co-located at the VA Bedford/VA Boston Healthcare Systems. As an applied medical anthropologist, she has almost two decades of experience conducting federally funded ethnographic research in healthcare settings. Her research focuses on the delivery of patient-centered care, particularly for people living with HIV. She is a fellow of the *Society for Applied Anthropology*.

Erin P. Finley is a Professor with the Departments of Medicine and Psychiatry and Behavioral Sciences at the Long School of Medicine, University of Texas (UT) Health San Antonio, and Core Investigator and Qualitative Methods Core Lead with the Center for the Study of Healthcare Innovation, Implementation, and Policy at the VA Greater Los Angeles Healthcare System. Her research interests include veterans' health, mental health, and diverse methods in implementation planning and evaluation.

Pragmatic Healthcare Ethnography

Methods to Study and Improve Healthcare

Alison B. Hamilton, Gemmae M. Fix and Erin P. Finley

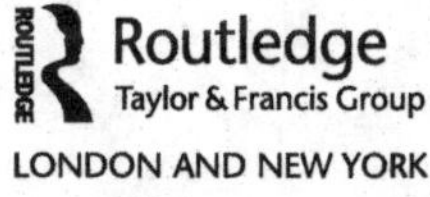

LONDON AND NEW YORK

Designed cover image: gremlin / Getty Images

First published 2025
by Routledge
4 Park Square, Milton Park, Abingdon, Oxon OX14 4RN

and by Routledge
605 Third Avenue, New York, NY 10158

Routledge is an imprint of the Taylor & Francis Group, an informa business

British Library Cataloguing-in-Publication Data
A catalogue record for this book is available from the British Library

ISBN: 978-1-032-48761-8 (hbk)
ISBN: 978-1-032-48760-1 (pbk)
ISBN: 978-1-003-39065-7 (ebk)

DOI: 10.4324/9781003390657

Typeset in Sabon
by KnowledgeWorks Global Ltd.

Alison dedicates this book to her children—Adesina, Negasi, and Bakari—who inspire her to dig as deep as possible to understand as much as possible.

Gemmae dedicates this book to her family (Eric, Zissa, Meyer, and Mom, Mimi), friends and nature—all of which bring her joy, awe, and gratitude.

Erin dedicates this book to her father, Dale Finley, who taught her about kindness, relationships, and respect.

Contents

List of figures and tables xi
About the authors xiii
Foreword by *David Atkins, MD, MPH* xv
Acknowledgments xxi
List of abbreviations xxiii

1 Pragmatic healthcare ethnography: An introduction 1
Setting the stage: Doing pragmatic healthcare ethnography 1
Introduction 2
Five central themes of ethnography 2
The importance of pragmatism 5
The authors as pragmatic ethnographers 5
Orientation to the book 6
Case 1: Thinking (and acting) ethnographically in VA healthcare research *(Heather Schacht Reisinger)* 6
Ethnography as a tool for change 7
Ethnographic epistemology in RAP 10
References 11

2 Designing ethnography for healthcare research 15
Introduction 15
When are ethnographic methods a good fit for healthcare research? 15
Methods: The building blocks of an ethnographic study design 18
Planning an ethnographic study 20
Sampling: Site and participant selection 23
A note about "N" *27*

Getting approval to conduct ethnography in healthcare settings 28
Is it research? *29*
Conclusion 33
Case 2: Designing an ethnographic evaluation for a substance use disorder intervention *(Megan McCullough)* 33
References 38

3 Conducting pragmatic ethnography in healthcare research **41**
Introduction 41
Where ethnography happens 41
Building ethnographic partnerships: Trust, reflexivity, and power 43
Observation 44
Fieldnotes and other methods of documenting observation *46*
Ethnographic interviews 50
Focus groups *52*
Patient and provider interviews *52*
Knowledge and expertise: Maintaining a beginner's mind *53*
Periodic reflections *53*
Team-based ethnography 55
Rapid, virtual, online, and video ethnographic approaches 57
Conclusion: Rigor, trustworthiness, and constraint 59
Case studies 3a and 3b: Participatory approaches in pragmatic healthcare ethnography 59
Case study 3a: Tending to partnerships *(Anaïs Tuepker)* 60
Case study 3b: Ethnography and participatory research: Bringing in community voices *(Gala True)* 63
References 68

4 Ethnography for understanding: Analytic approaches **73**
Selecting and applying analytic strategies and tools 73
Approaching the data 74
Getting organized *75*
Getting familiar *75*
Getting strategic *76*
Using tools: Memoing 77
Methods memos *77*
Research question memo *77*
Emergent discoveries memo *78*
Future studies memo *78*
Episode profiles *79*
Topic memos *80*
Using tools: Diagramming, visual displays, and analytic templates 81
Using tools: Coding 85
Synthesizing for holistic understanding 88
Conclusion: Rigorous pragmatic ethnography 88
Case 4: Visibility and participation in ethnographic analysis *(Sarah Ono)* 90
References 92

5 Sharing ethnographic findings **97**
Introduction 97
Getting started: What do we want to share? 97
Building on our data sources and analytic resources 99
Reaching our target audience(s) 100
Selecting journals and publishing ethnographic work *100*
Presenting ethnographic work to academic audiences *103*
Preparing nonacademic products *103*
Demonstrating rigor 106
Ethics: Protecting research participants 108
Case 5: Creating space for transparency and dialogue to improve data accuracy and tailored dissemination of ethnographic data *(Justeen Hyde)* 109
Local Whole Health leaders 113
Office of Patient-Centered Care and Cultural Transformation (OPCC&CT) 114
Congress 114
Conclusions 115
References 115

6 Crafting a new ethnography **119**
Introduction 119
New opportunities for ethnographic theory and methods 119
Ethnography as part of learning healthcare systems 121
References 122

Afterword *by Annette Boaz, PhD* **123**
Index **127**

Figures and tables

Figures

2.1 Compassionate relationship-centered care: Being recognized—Alex's story 36
2.2 Compassionate relationship-centered care: Knowing the little things—Sandra's story 37
2.3 Compassionate relationship-centered care: Making time—Scott's story 37
4.1 Moving from research question to data analysis and understanding 74
4.2 Qualitative data collection spectrum 76
4.3 Sample diagram of life history trajectories (Hamilton and Goeders 2010) 82
4.4 Sample "timeline map" for visualizing mixed-method data (Reproduced with permission from Brunner et al. 2022) 83
4.5 Sample composites summarizing distinct features of patient experience—Ernest 85
4.6 Sample composites summarizing distinct features of patient experience—Daniel 86
4.7 Sample composites summarizing distinct features of patient experience—Carl 86
5.1 Thinking through sharing ethnographic findings 98
5.2 Summary for patient advisory groups 105
5.3 Paper draft in progress using data to support the narrative 107
5.4 VA's conceptual model of Whole Health 109
5.5 Whole Health system of care 111

Tables

2.1 Questions to consider when deciding whether ethnography is appropriate for a given study 16
2.2 A brief overview of common methods in ethnographic studies 18
2.3 Example patient data collection plan (Fix 2008) 20
2.4 Example of study participants (Fix 2008) 20
2.5 Considerations when planning an ethnographic study design 21

2.6 Study design overview template 21
2.7 Example study overview 22
2.8 Data summary template 23
2.9 Example data summary for a study of implementing evidence-based practices for women veterans in VA health care (Hamilton et al. 2023) 24
2.10 Ethnographic features 34
3.1 Common roles on an ethnographic team 56
4.1 Example data spreadsheet 75
4.2 Common types of memos in pragmatic analysis 77
4.3 Sample brief summary of life history information 81
4.4 Sample analytic synthesis template 84
5.1 Team composition and clinician conceptualization of patient behavior (Fix et al. 2018) 100
5.2 Audiences and common products for ethnographic findings 104

About the authors

Alison B. Hamilton is a VA Research Career Scientist and Implementation Research Director with the Center for the Study of Healthcare Innovation, Implementation, and Policy at the VA Greater Los Angeles Healthcare System; a Professor-in-Residence in the University of California Los Angeles (UCLA) Department of Psychiatry and Biobehavioral Science, David Geffen School of Medicine; and an Honorary Professor in the Department of Psychiatry and Mental Health, University of Cape Town, South Africa. Her research interests include gender and health, mental health, implementation science, and research methods.

Gemmae M. Fix is an Associate Professor at Boston University Chobanian & Avedisian School of Medicine and a Research Health Scientist with the Center for Healthcare Organization and Implementation Research, co-located at the VA Bedford/VA Boston Healthcare Systems. As an applied medical anthropologist, she has almost two decades of experience conducting federally funded ethnographic research in healthcare settings. Her research focuses on the delivery of patient-centered care, particularly for people living with HIV. She is a fellow of the *Society for Applied Anthropology*.

Erin P. Finley is a Professor with the Departments of Medicine and Psychiatry and Behavioral Sciences at the Long School of Medicine, University of Texas (UT) Health San Antonio, and Core Investigator and Qualitative Methods Core Lead with the Center for the Study of Healthcare Innovation, Implementation, and Policy at the VA Greater Los Angeles Healthcare System. Her research interests include veterans' health, mental health, and diverse methods in implementation planning and evaluation.

Foreword

David Atkins, MD, MPH

The quest to improve health care in the United States has been a frustrating mix of breakthroughs, misplaced priorities, and persisting problems. Amazing advances have revolutionized treatments for certain cancers, cystic fibrosis, and obesity, while we continue to lag other Western countries in most health outcomes and exhibit persistent disparities along lines of race, ethnicity, and geography. Despite being an outlier in terms of healthcare spending, the US lags 38 other high-income countries in life expectancy (Gunja, Gumas, and Williams 2023). Experts have attributed these problems to a range of issues, including income inequality, systemic racism, gaps in healthcare coverage, our disorganized system of health care, and profit-driven private healthcare.

The US Department of Veteran Affairs (VA) healthcare system, where I worked for 15 years as the Director of Health Services Research and Development, is an interesting laboratory of what is possible in a system free of the uniquely American problems of high insurance costs, homelessness, perverse financial incentives, and a fragmented care system. The VA cares for more than 9 million veterans ("About the Veterans Health Administration" 2023). Structural advantages have helped VA achieve population-level outcomes that are generally superior to those in the private sector (Kizer and Dudley 2009; Apaydin et al. 2023; O'Hanlon et al. 2017). Nonetheless, 30 years of health services research have revealed a number of lessons: variation in quality is a persistent problem even in a national system with good data; change is slow and hard; coordinating care for patients with complex comorbidities is difficult; and creating a truly patient-centered approach to health and health care remains an aspirational goal.

In the United States, we can create amazing treatment advances, but we are far from consistently getting the right treatment to the right patient at the right time. A 2005 paper pointed out that ensuring all eligible patients got recommended therapies was more useful than improving the efficacy of those treatments (Woolf 2005). Most of the billions of private and public biomedical investments continue to be made in improving treatments rather than improving the delivery of our existing therapies. Even when we focus on how to get the right treatments to the right patient, much of the attention is on technological approaches like artificial intelligence (AI), machine learning, and genomics. These approaches ignore that health care at its core is a social process involving a web of complex human interactions—between clinicians and their patients, among members of a healthcare team, between managers and staff, and among patients and their caregivers. We cannot achieve the "quadruple aim" of high-quality, high-value, equitable, and patient-centered care without understanding the human actions and interactions that influence the behaviors of patients, clinicians, managers, and families (Bodenheimer and Sinsky 2014).

The VA has been a leading home for health services research in the United States. Relative to other large health systems, the VA benefits from a Congressionally appropriated research budget, robust clinical data drawing on a three-decade-old electronic health record, and a community of embedded intramural researchers at over 100 medical centers. VA researchers work closely with VA patients and clinicians, and over half of VA-funded principal investigators are practicing VA clinicians themselves. At the heart of this effort are the patients who participate in research out of their commitment to helping improve care for their fellow veterans (Hyde et al. 2018). Health services research in VA is a $120 million program involving over 300 active projects, 22 research centers, and over 1,000 MD and PhD researchers. As a physician, I came to especially value the contribution of the diverse community of non-physician researchers, including epidemiologists, biostatisticians, psychologists, economists, sociologists, and anthropologists. The unique advantage of VA research is our ability to conduct mixed-methods research that combines quantitative and qualitative methods to identify quality gaps, understand contributing factors, design interventions to address these gaps, and test these interventions in the real world.

During my tenure in VA, as we worked to bring our research into closer collaboration with the leaders of VA's clinical programs, I came to realize that our partners rarely needed help from researchers to learn "what" was happening in their programs. Many of VA's clinical programs have sophisticated teams that track and analyze the delivery and outcomes of care, reporting numerous quality metrics at the level of medical centers, clinics, and individual clinicians. Partners did need our help, however, to know the "why" of what was happening: why did certain veteran groups lag in certain outcomes or how did certain medical centers excel in rolling out new programs? As one example, we have known for some time that Black veterans are less likely than white veterans to receive and continue long-term medication-assisted therapy (MAT) for opioid use disorder (Manhapra, Quinones, and Rosenheck 2016; Priest et al. 2022), but we needed research to untangle the why. Was the disparity due to greater barriers to accessing the drugs, problems adhering to requirements for MAT programs, or skepticism in some communities about long-term medications for substance use disorders? As Drs. Alison Hamilton, Gemmae Fix, and Erin Finley and their contributors highlight throughout this book, qualitative—moreover, ethnographic—methods are ideally suited to address "why" questions (Husain et al. 2023; Madden 2019).

The VA has proven to be a great home for anthropologists to contribute to healthcare research. Anthropologists have been critical in bringing rigorous methods to study the behaviors of patients, caregivers, and members of the VA healthcare system. At last count, the anthropology community of practice in VA had 150 members! A survey of VA anthropologists indicated that their most common research areas included implementation science, quality improvement, mental health, and access to care (Fix et al. 2023). Implementation science has emerged as an area where VA health services research has been a national leader, catalyzed by the 25-year-old Quality Enhancement Research Initiative (QUERI) program (Kilbourne et al. 2019). Funded by the clinical budget, QUERI engages researchers to help VA implement and scale up new programs and quality improvement efforts. Among recent high-profile programs benefiting from QUERI and the anthropologists working with QUERI have been the national implementation of patient-aligned care teams (VA's medical home) (Tuepker et al. 2014), growth and improvement of women's health services (Hamilton et al. 2017), and expansion of MAT (Hawkins et al. 2021). Several of these anthropologists have contributed to this book.

Ethnographic research is an important component of the qualitative research conducted in VA. Due to specific eligibility requirements for VA care, the VA patient population has a disproportionate number of patients who have complex co-morbidities and complicating social situations. Almost half of the six million veterans seen in any year have at least one mental health diagnosis; most are older, and many live alone. The VA has expanded its caregiver programs, recognizing the need to support family caregivers who are critical to enabling veterans to be cared for at home. By collecting detailed data on the lived experiences of patients, caregivers, and members of healthcare teams, ethnography can help illustrate what is needed to truly provide patient-centered, coordinated care for complex patients. Pragmatic ethnographic research can identify unique barriers to care, problems in communication and coordination within the healthcare team, and obstacles to implementing new models of care. A truism of the VA health system is that what works in Albuquerque doesn't necessarily work in Albany—and ethnographic methods help us understand those contextual factors.

There are specific reasons why pragmatic ethnographic research will remain important to VA. Moreover, since the challenges facing VA are representative of larger national trends, the value of ethnographers should be true for all large healthcare organizations within the United States and beyond.

First, complexity is the rule rather than the exception in health care. Complex patients account for the majority of healthcare spending in the US. In the VA, it is not uncommon for a single patient to have multiple "care coordinators," each in charge of specific issues such as women's health or suicide prevention. As the population ages and problems with addiction and mental health grow, we need a better understanding of how teams operate and communicate with each other.

Second, the VA goal of "Whole Health" rests on putting the patient at the center of care and is grounded in the patient's life experiences and goals (Krist, South-Paul, and Meisnere 2023). Achieving "patient-centeredness" requires a cultural transformation, predicated on understanding what that looks like to patients and how to support teams of doctors, nurses, pharmacists, mental health providers, and staff to provide it. Gemmae and contributing author Justeen Hyde are central to this work, helping VA identify key aspects needed for system change (Bokhour et al. 2022; Fix et al. 2018).

Third, VA has a long-standing commitment to health equity. Ethnography can help us to understand the cultural forces (for patients and providers) that contribute to inequity and can in turn inform interventions. For example, building on her ethnographic work on serious mental illness among African Caribbeans (Eliacin 2013), anthropologist Johanne Eliacin conducted extensive qualitative research on racial disparities in mental health treatment and outcomes among veterans (Eliacin et al. 2021). She then developed a peer-led patient navigation program to improve racially diverse veterans' engagement in mental health services (Eliacin et al. 2023a, 2023b). Her intervention is grounded in an understanding of patients' social contexts and the patient-clinician relationship.

Finally, healthcare systems need effective partnerships between researchers and clinical partners (Atkins, Kullgren, and Simpson 2021). Even in VA, where these partnerships are the norm, the biggest barrier remains a cultural one due to the differing expectations, priorities, incentives, and constraints of the research and practice communities. Alison and her team's work on harassment—which won the VA Health Services Research Health Systems Impact Award—illustrates what can happen when partnerships are effective, drawing on rich, multimethod research evidence, public engagement, and policy change to address a high-priority issue (Fenwick et al. 2021; Dyer et al. 2021).

Those engaged in pragmatic healthcare ethnography should remain alert to some specific challenges if they want their work to be valued and supported more broadly. First, as a therapist colleague reminded me, "insight is overrated." To truly be of value, ethnographers need to turn their insights into recommendations for action or tools to help the people trying to understand and foster change; this is the pragmatic angle that Alison, Gemmae, and Erin advance in this book. Second, they need to broaden the audience for their message beyond academic researchers, as the authors explain in Chapter 5. This may require translating academic jargon into concepts that busy clinicians and managers or facility leaders can understand. Finally, they need to draw upon more rapid methods to provide useful insights—methods that align with the pace of change in clinical care rather than the multi-year funding of research grants. This book provides practical strategies to address these challenges.

In closing, change is hard, is often resisted, and the results of change may appear relatively modest and slow. But the core of a "learning healthcare system" is the ability to continually examine and evolve to deliver care that is more consistent, higher quality, more aligned with patient values, and higher value. Analytics may identify areas where change is needed, but pragmatic ethnographic methods are essential for understanding what change really involves and how to make it a reality.

References

"About the Veterans Health Administration." 2023. November 8, 2023. https://www.va.gov/health/aboutvha.asp.

Apaydin, Eric A., Neil M. Paige, Meron M. Begashaw, Jody Larkin, Isomi M. Miake-Lye, and Paul G. Shekelle. 2023. "Veterans Health Administration (VA) vs. Non-VA Healthcare Quality: A Systematic Review." *Journal of General Internal Medicine* 38 (9): 2179–88. https://doi.org/10.1007/s11606-023-08207-2.

Atkins, David, Jeffrey T. Kullgren, and Lisa Simpson. 2021. "Enhancing the Role of Research in a Learning Health Care System." *Healthcare* 8 (June): 100556. https://doi.org/10.1016/j.hjdsi.2021.100556.

Bodenheimer, Thomas, and Christine Sinsky. 2014. "From Triple to Quadruple Aim: Care of the Patient Requires Care of the Provider." *The Annals of Family Medicine* 12 (6): 573–76. https://doi.org/10.1370/afm.1713.

Bokhour, Barbara G., Justeen Hyde, Benjamin Kligler, Hannah Gelman, Lauren Gaj, Anna M. Barker, Jamie Douglas, Rian DeFaccio, Stephanie L. Taylor, and Steven B. Zeliadt. 2022. "From Patient Outcomes to System Change: Evaluating the Impact of VHA's Implementation of the Whole Health System of Care." *Health Services Research* 57 (S1): 53–65. https://doi.org/10.1111/1475-6773.13938.

Dyer, Karen E., Alison B. Hamilton, Elizabeth M. Yano, Jessica L. Moreau, Susan M. Frayne, Diane V. Carney, Rachel E. Golden, and Ruth Klap. 2021. "Mobilizing Embedded Research and Operations Partnerships to Address Harassment of Women Veterans at VA Medical Facilities." *Healthcare* 8 (June): 100513. https://doi.org/10.1016/j.hjdsi.2020.100513.

Eliacin, Johanne. 2013. "Social Capital, Narratives of Fragmentation, and Schizophrenia: An Ethnographic Exploration of Factors Shaping African-Caribbeans' Social Capital and Mental Health in a North London Community." *Culture, Medicine, and Psychiatry* 37 (3): 465–87. https://doi.org/10.1007/s11013-013-9322-2.

Eliacin, Johanne, Marianne S. Matthias, Diana J. Burgess, Scott Patterson, Teresa Damush, Mandi Pratt-Chapman, Mark McGovern, et al. 2021. "Pre-Implementation Evaluation of PARTNER-MH: A Mental Healthcare Disparity Intervention for Minority Veterans in the VHA." *Administration and Policy in Mental Health and Mental Health Services Research* 48 (1): 46–60. https://doi.org/10.1007/s10488-020-01048-9.

Eliacin, Johanne, Diana Burgess, Angela L Rollins, Scott Patterson, Teresa Damush, Matthew J Bair, Michelle P Salyers, et al. 2023. "Outcomes of a Peer-Led Navigation Program, PARTNER-MH, for Racially Minoritized Veterans Receiving Mental Health Services: A Pilot Randomized Controlled Trial to Assess Feasibility and Acceptability." *Translational Behavioral Medicine* 13 (9): 710–21. https://doi.org/10.1093/tbm/ibad027.

Eliacin, Johanne, Marianne S. Matthias, Kenzie A. Cameron, and Diana J. Burgess. 2023. "Veterans' Views of PARTNER-MH, a Peer-Led Patient Navigation Intervention, to Improve Patient Engagement in Care and Patient-Clinician Communication: A Qualitative Study." *Patient Education and Counseling* 114 (September): 107847. https://doi.org/10.1016/j.pec.2023.107847.

Fenwick, Karissa M., Rachel E. Golden, Susan M. Frayne, Alison B. Hamilton, Elizabeth M. Yano, Diane V. Carney, and Ruth Klap. 2021. "Women Veterans' Experiences of Harassment and Perceptions of Veterans Affairs Health Care Settings during a National Anti-Harassment Campaign." *Women's Health Issues* 31 (6): 567–75. https://doi.org/10.1016/j.whi.2021.06.005.

Fix, Gemmae M., Carol VanDeusen Lukas, Rendelle E. Bolton, Jennifer N. Hill, Nora Mueller, Sherri L. LaVela, and Barbara G. Bokhour. 2018. "Patient-centred Care Is a Way of Doing Things: How Healthcare Employees Conceptualize Patient-centred Care." *Health Expectations* 21 (1): 300–7. https://doi.org/10.1111/hex.12615.

Fix, Gemmae, Aaron Seaman, Linda Nichols, Sarah Ono, Nicholas Rattray, Samantha Solimeo, Heather Schacht Reisinger, and Traci Abraham. 2023. "Building a Community of Anthropological Practice: The Case of Anthropologists Working within the United States' Largest Health Care System." *Human Organization* 82 (2): 169–81. https://doi.org/10.17730/1938-3525-82.2.169.

Gunja, Munira Z., Evan D. Gumas, and Reginald D. Williams. 2023. "U.S. Health Care from a Global Perspective, 2022: *Accelerating Spending, Worsening Outcomes.*" *The Commonwealth Fund*. https://www.commonwealthfund.org/publications/issue-briefs/2023/jan/us-health-care-global-perspective-2022.

Hamilton, Alison B., Julian Brunner, Cindy Cain, Emmeline Chuang, Tana M. Luger, Ismelda Canelo, Lisa Rubenstein, and Elizabeth M. Yano. 2017. "Engaging Multilevel Stakeholders in an Implementation Trial of Evidence-Based Quality Improvement in VA Women's Health Primary Care." *Translational Behavioral Medicine* 7 (3): 478–85. https://doi.org/10.1007/s13142-017-0501-5.

Hawkins, Eric J., Anissa N. Danner, Carol A. Malte, Brittany E. Blanchard, Emily C. Williams, Hildi J. Hagedorn, Adam J. Gordon, et al. 2021. "Clinical Leaders and Providers' Perspectives on Delivering Medications for the Treatment of Opioid Use Disorder in Veteran Affairs' Facilities." *Addiction Science & Clinical Practice* 16 (1): 55. https://doi.org/10.1186/s13722-021-00263-5.

Husain, Jawad M., Devin Cromartie, Emma Fitzelle-Jones, Annelise Brochier, Christina P.C. Borba, and Cristina Montalvo. 2023. "A Qualitative Analysis of Barriers to Opioid Agonist Treatment for Racial/Ethnic Minoritized Populations." *Journal of Substance Abuse Treatment* 144 (January): 108918. https://doi.org/10.1016/j.jsat.2022.108918.

Hyde, Justeen K., Leah Wendleton, Kelty Fehling, Jeff Whittle, Gala True, Alison Hamilton, Jennifer M. Gierisch, et al. 2018. "Strengthening Excellence in Research through Veteran Engagement (SERVE): Toolkit for Veteran Engagement in Research (Version 1)." Veterans Health Administration, Health Services Research and Development. https://www.hsrd.research.va.gov/for_researchers/serve/

Kilbourne, Amy M., David E. Goodrich, Isomi Miake-Lye, Melissa Z. Braganza, and Nicholas W. Bowersox. 2019. "Quality Enhancement Research Initiative Implementation Roadmap: Toward Sustainability of Evidence-Based Practices in a Learning Health System." *Medical Care* 57 (Suppl 3): S286–93. https://doi.org/10.1097/MLR.0000000000001144.

Kizer, Kenneth W., and R. Adams Dudley. 2009. "Extreme Makeover: Transformation of the Veterans Health Care System." *Annual Review of Public Health* 30: 313–39.

Krist, Alex H., Jeannette E. South-Paul, and Marc Meisnere. 2023. "Achieving Whole Health for Veterans and the Nation: A National Academies of Sciences, Engineering, and Medicine Report." *JAMA Health Forum* 4 (5): e230874. https://doi.org/10.1001/jamahealthforum.2023.0874.

Madden, Erin Fanning. 2019. "Intervention Stigma: How Medication-Assisted Treatment Marginalizes Patients and Providers." *Social Science & Medicine* 232 (July): 324–31. https://doi.org/10.1016/j.socscimed.2019.05.02.

Manhapra, Ajay, Lantie Quinones, and Robert Rosenheck. 2016. "Characteristics of Veterans Receiving Buprenorphine vs. Methadone for Opioid Use Disorder Nationally in the Veterans Health Administration." *Drug and Alcohol Dependence* 160 (March): 82–89. https://doi.org/10.1016/j.drugalcdep.2015.12.035.

O'Hanlon, Claire, Christina Huang, Elizabeth Sloss, Rebecca Anhang Price, Peter Hussey, Carrie Farmer, and Courtney Gidengil. 2017. "Comparing VA and Non-VA Quality of Care: A Systematic Review." *Journal of General Internal Medicine* 32 (1): 105–21. https://doi.org/10.1007/s11606-016-3775-2.

Priest, Kelsey C., Caroline A. King, Honora Englander, Travis I. Lovejoy, and Dennis McCarty. 2022. "Differences in the Delivery of Medications for Opioid Use Disorder during Hospitalization by Racial Categories: A Retrospective Cohort Analysis;" *Substance Abuse* 43 (1): 1251–59. https://doi.org/10.1080/08897077.2022.2074601.

Tuepker, Anaïs, Devan Kansagara, Eleni Skaperdas, Christina Nicolaidis, Sandra Joos, Michael Alperin, and David Hickam. 2014. "'We've Not Gotten Even Close to What We Want to Do': A Qualitative Study of Early Patient-Centered Medical Home Implementation." *Journal of General Internal Medicine* 29 (S2): 614–22. https://doi.org/10.1007/s11606-013-2690-z.

Woolf, Steven H. 2005. "The Break-Even Point: When Medical Advances Are Less Important Than Improving the Fidelity with Which They Are Delivered." *The Annals of Family Medicine* 3 (6): 545–52. https://doi.org/10.1370/afm.406.

Acknowledgments

We would like to thank our VA colleagues, specifically our contributors, who challenge us to learn, innovate, and grow. They have been brilliant collaborators for years and encouraged us to bring this book to fruition. Their case studies fulfill our vision not only to articulate but also to illustrate rich, impactful, pragmatic approaches to healthcare ethnography. We would also like to acknowledge Dr. Svea Closser for her invaluable review of an early draft.

Alison would like to acknowledge Dr. Doug Hollan, for teaching and mentoring her in all things ethnographic and person-centered; Dr. Ray Maietta, for engaging in an enriching qualitative methods journey with her for over two decades; and her parents, Dr. Stanley Hamilton and Hilary Hamilton, for giving her a love of learning and a passion for health and health care.

Gemmae would like to acknowledge the broader community of social scientists, many of whom she came to know through the *Society for Applied Anthropology*. This community both inspires and drives her work. It's these relationships that make that work meaningful.

Erin would like to acknowledge Dr. Peter J. Brown for being a steadfast mentor and amplifier to a generation of Emory anthropologists, and for role-modeling such a rich and meaningful life. She would also like to thank her family, for all of the support and all of the joy. India, Ivan, Lorenzo, Marco, and Stefano—you are cherished!

Abbreviations

CARA	Comprehensive Addictions and Recovery Act
CPP	clinical pharmacy practitioner
CPT	cognitive processing therapy
CRVA-SUD	Clinical Pharmacy Practitioners for Rural Veteran Access: Substance Use Disorder
EBP	evidence-based practice
EBQI	Evidence-Based Quality Improvement
HIV	human immunodeficiency virus
IRB	Institutional Review Board
MHV	My Healthe*e*Vet
OPCC&CT	Office of Patient-Centered Care & Cultural Transformation
PACT	Patient-Aligned Care Teams
PAR	participatory action research
PE	prolonged exposure
PTSD	post-traumatic stress disorder
QUERI	Quality Enhancement Research Initiative
RAP	Rapid Assessment Process
REM	Ripple Effects Mapping
REP	Replicating Effective Programs
TBI	traumatic brain injury
TOP	Telemedicine Outreach for PTSD
TTP	Tending to Partnerships
VA	Veterans Health Administration
VISION	Veteran-Informed Safety Intervention and Outreach Network
VPC	Veteran Peer Champion
VSO	Veteran Service Organization

CHAPTER 1

Pragmatic healthcare ethnography

An introduction

Ethnography means "to write people." A research method used to explore cultural phenomena, ethnography dates back to the 1920s and even earlier. Ethnography provides a useful set of tools for observing how people act in the world, helps us understand why people act as they do, and generates a holistic perspective on the topic under study. Ethnographic methods help document the difference between what people say and what they do, and they attend to environment and group dynamics. Ethnography can be challenging to integrate into rapidly paced projects because it can be time-intensive (and therefore costly) in both data collection and analysis. In this chapter, we provide an introduction to ethnography, offer some guidance on why ethnography matters in healthcare research, and outline our approach to pragmatic healthcare ethnography. A case study illustrates how ethnography can be used as a tool for change.

Setting the stage: Doing pragmatic healthcare ethnography

Gemmae Fix, an anthropologist and one of the authors of this book, was faced with the challenge of understanding variations in care for people with human immunodeficiency virus (HIV) across a health system. To better understand this problem, Gemmae not only interviewed 30 providers but also observed 43 clinical encounters and conducted an additional 30 clinic observations across eight HIV practices. By "being there" in the practices, she was able to observe how providers were talking about *and to* patients, which revealed that providers had attitudes toward patients within a moral framework. Those who thought about their patients as "good"/adherent patients versus "bad"/non-compliant patients tended to miss factors within patients' lives that may have contributed to non-optimal health behaviors and poor health outcomes. In contrast, providers who conceptualized patients' health behaviors within their socio-cultural environments (e.g., housing, employment) thought about patients' unique needs in the context of their lives. This latter perspective did not ascribe moral judgments to difficult or non-adherent behaviors but rather contextualized them. Understanding patients as people within their

DOI: 10.4324/9781003390657-1

daily lives facilitated care that matched patients' needs, epitomizing patient-centered care. Had Gemmae and her team only relied on interviews with providers, the dynamics and organizational context of care for patients living with HIV would not have been captured. As they note, "*We saw care planning happening within a context of what the clinic could offer.*" This ethnographic case study was conducted over one year of a three-year study, by busy researchers, in the context of busy clinics, with busy providers. This work is emblematic of the type of pragmatic healthcare ethnography that we describe in this book.

Introduction

Ethnography means "to write people." A research method used to explore cultural phenomena holistically, ethnography dates back to the 1920s and even earlier. Ethnography refers both to something you do—a process—and something you produce (an ethnography) (Box 1.1). It emphasizes seeking to understand insider ("emic") perspectives on a phenomenon or problem and assumes that people's beliefs, behaviors, and relationships are important to understand in their unique contexts (i.e., cultural relativism). Ethnography typically draws upon multiple methods, including but not limited to qualitative methods (particularly observation), to explore these insider perspectives, with attention to the ethnographer's positionality. It is carried out in "natural" settings, that is, the ethnographer goes to (or works/lives in) the setting(s) where the phenomenon of interest is occurring and observes naturally occurring behaviors and interactions. These natural settings are different from settings where people are gathered explicitly for the purposes of research. Traditional ethnography is known for being time-intensive and longitudinal, with ethnographers often spending lengthy periods of time in "the field" (i.e., the site(s) of research) and returning year after year to develop deeper, holistic understanding (Bernard 2018). Perhaps due to this reputation and the skills needed to conduct ethnographic research, ethnography has not been a go-to method in healthcare research. However, a growing body of ethnographic work illustrates that ethnography can and should be used in healthcare-related research to generate deeper, contextualized understandings of health, health care, and health outcomes (Black et al. 2021; Dixon-Woods 2003; Savage 2006).

Five central themes of ethnography

Ethnography provides a useful set of tools for observing how people act in the world and helping us to understand why people act as they do. Ethnographic methods help to document the difference between what people say and what they do while attending to

Box 1.1 Defining ethnography

Emic, insider perspectives
Aim of holistic understanding
Emphasis on cultural relativism
More than one method, often including observation
Often longitudinal
Recognition of the researcher's positionality

Box 1.2 Five central themes of ethnography

Ethnography features lived experiences.
Ethnography is inherently holistic.
Ethnography is concerned with power.
Ethnography entails reflexivity.
Ethnography requires flexibility.

the environment and group dynamics. Throughout this book, we will refer to five central themes in ethnography that are particularly relevant to healthcare research (Box 1.2).

First, *ethnography features lived experiences*. When ethnographers spend time in the field, they do so to be surrounded by day-to-day life and to experience life in the setting of interest. In healthcare-related ethnography, this could mean spending time in a healthcare setting and/or with people where they are experiencing their health conditions (at home, at work, in their communities). It could also mean spending time where people are trained to become healthcare providers. Fundamentally, this "time spent" provides opportunities for ethnographers to see what is happening in the environment, as people are living their lives and engaging in day-to-day activities. This engagement often means getting and staying out of the way, so the ethnographer's presence minimally disrupts the usual flow of activities. Observational methods (e.g., participant observation, direct observation) are a common tool of ethnographers. They can reveal critical information that would not be accessible with other types of data collection (Fix et al. 2022). For example, to better understand self-management of diabetes, Hinder and Greenhalgh (2012) interviewed and spent time with people with diabetes in their homes and communities. They were able to see how people were able (or unable) to accomplish self-management tasks within their everyday lives and observed that non-engagement with self-management is more than an individual issue—it is relational and social, with practice and policy implications.

Second, *ethnography is inherently holistic,* acknowledging the relationship between isolated elements of any system and the broader whole. For example, individual experiences of illness are profoundly shaped by the larger social, cultural, and structural environments, including local understandings of health, policy, and economic factors shaping access to care, and so on. Similarly, care practices in a given clinic are likely to be shaped by the prior training and experience of individual providers, clinical practice guidelines, the standards and requirements of the larger healthcare organization in which the clinic is embedded, and/or relevant state and federal insurance policies (e.g., formulary restrictions). *Seeking holistic understanding means understanding how these varied parts come together to shape patterns of behavior and experience, which—in the context of pragmatic healthcare ethnography—can in turn support developing innovative solutions for improvement.* Understanding how patients are experiencing a particular appointment scheduling system, or how providers struggle to enact an overly complex workflow, can inform creating more intuitive processes, reducing complexity, or facilitating richer communication.

Alongside this holistic focus comes an appreciation for how theory can help to make sense of the patterns we observe, and how ethnography can help to refine and generate theory. By "theory," we are referring to an organizing way of understanding a phenomenon. Because ethnography is concerned with why and how people do what they do, theory can help with developing ideas, guiding data collection, understanding perspectives, and interpreting data. In applied healthcare research, we have theories about many phenomena, such as what predicts outcomes, how interventions work, how policy is enacted, and how people and organizations behave and change in relation to health and health care.

Third, *ethnography is concerned with power*. The ethnographic lens assumes that power is inherent to human behavior and how we relate to one another. Power is everywhere, seen and unseen, and the settings where we conduct ethnography have power "baked in" to social relationships and structures (Finley et al. 2023). Some data collection methods, such as interviews, are limited in their potential to reveal power dynamics, which are often enacted and unconscious rather than verbalized and conscious. In ethnographic work, by situating ourselves in healthcare settings, we may observe power in many forms, including not only how people interact but also how space is designed and how people move through and use space. Building on the example of Gemmae's work at the beginning of this chapter, by being there she could observe the power dynamics in the clinical encounter. She observed an HIV provider talk to a person living with HIV about being a "good patient." By speaking to the patient like a child, the provider effectively stopped any communication about why the patient might have been having difficulty managing his HIV medications.

Fourth, *ethnography entails reflexivity*, that is, being aware of and documenting your identities, role(s), presence, actions, and feelings (Davis and Breede 2015). Historically, there was a notion of going into the field "tabula rasa," ostensibly knowing very little and developing an understanding from the "ground up," by virtue of time spent and iterative data collection during that time spent. However, critical scholarship has debunked this notion, pointing out that our positionality as the instrument of data collection is never neutral, and that we need to be as aware and transparent as possible about our assumptions and biases going into the field (Knauft 1996; Trundle and Phillips 2023). We are not neutral, but rather are actively engaged in making sense of what we are seeing, hearing, observing, sensing, and thinking. In applied healthcare research, we are typically quite knowledgeable about our research topics—including our theoretical lens—as we likely had to convey that knowledge in order to generate a compelling research question and receive funding for the research. Furthermore, time for the research is typically limited and concentrated, which can hamper more exploratory research. *We find in pragmatic healthcare ethnography that it is essential to articulate what we think we know prior to the ethnography, to be open to learning and recognizing what we don't know as we conduct the ethnography, and to reflect on what we learned versus what we thought we knew before we conducted the research*. Snell-Rood and colleagues (2021) point out the importance of remaining open to *emergence*. In other words, we are not embarking on ethnography to prove that what we know is correct, but rather to discover what we did not know and more about what we thought we knew.

Finally, and of particular relevance to pragmatic ethnography, *ethnography requires flexibility*. Given that this methodology entails being in natural settings—settings that were not constructed for research—it is critical that we remain open to changing dynamics, shifting methods, expanding or contracting the sampling frame, and refining the research questions, all of which we address in this book. Human behavior—including health behavior—is unpredictable and nonlinear. Ethnography too is unpredictable and nonlinear: our plan for a day in the field may change for a variety of reasons, some of which will be driven by what we are learning, and some of which will be driven by dynamics well outside of our control.

The importance of pragmatism

This book is about "pragmatic healthcare ethnography." We situate this type of ethnography within a growing trend in healthcare research to embrace pragmatism, which means "keeping our focus on issues and data relevant for making decisions and taking action" (Glasgow 2013). Conducting ethnography in healthcare settings and other health-related environments requires pragmatism, as our research is typically being done for practical reasons, in environments that are busy, dynamic, and complex (Morgan-Trimmer and Wood 2016). As the contributions of this approach become more widely embraced (Cubellis et al. 2021; Gertner et al. 2021), and as more social scientists enter into the field of applied healthcare research, an increasing number of tailored ethnographic approaches are being developed, such as rapid ethnography (Palinkas and Zatzick 2019; Vindrola-Padros and Vindrola-Padros 2018), focused ethnography (Bikker et al. 2017), applied ethnography (Savage 2006), and video (Neuwirth et al. 2012) and video-reflexive ethnography (Ajjawi et al. 2020). Consistent with these approaches, we emphasize *feasibility*, taking time constraints and team-based data collection and analysis into consideration.

The authors as pragmatic ethnographers

The three of us authors are anthropologists, and we have all conducted pragmatic healthcare ethnographies across a variety of healthcare settings, including primary care and mental health clinics, surgical units, HIV clinics, community-based substance abuse treatment clinics, and people's homes (Finley 2011; Fix et al. 2018; Hamilton 2012). We each found our way to healthcare ethnography as part of a search to better understand the nature of healing and distress, with key moments lighting the way. For Alison, it was talking with women in Trinidad and Tobago about appreciating life, family, and natural beauty while also hearing about struggles, limited resources, and ailments; sitting in a treatment clinic in Hawaii, learning about how crystal methamphetamine "hit" the state in the 1980s due to its geographic position between Asian methamphetamine markets and the US mainland, devasting communities across generations; interviewing a woman in a residential treatment program and hearing about how she desperately sought prenatal care but was turned away repeatedly from services because she was "just a strung-out meth addict" who was told she "didn't care" about potentially harming her fetus. For Gemmae, her curiosity, pragmatism, and flexibility led to a dissertation that explored patients' experiences after open heart surgery. She visited these patients in their homes, met their families, and followed them for several months after their surgeries. This window into patients' lives was in stark contrast to providers who characterized recovery as "when the patient goes home." For Erin, it was sitting with a former soldier in a café in Jerusalem, listening as he described what it felt like to lead a military unit at 19; watching a mother silently give birth in a midwife's home in Guatemala, too wary of the hospital to go there; leaning against a methadone clinic reception desk to hear the news after the second plane hit the World Trade Center on 9/11; the broadcast interspersed with the conversation of two women who had recently lost a friend to overdose. Much of our work has been conducted in a US-based integrated healthcare system, the Veterans Health Administration (VA), which provides a shared context for many of the examples we provide. In this book, we draw upon our experiences to convey core principles for conducting pragmatic healthcare ethnography, as well as offering insights into the many emerging approaches and how they can be used to strengthen and extend applied healthcare research.

Orientation to the book

In this book, we provide pragmatic guidance on why ethnography matters in applied healthcare research and how to incorporate it into this type of research, which encompasses health services and implementation research. In each chapter, we provide an overview of key principles for conducting ethnography in healthcare settings, inclusive of community-based settings (i.e., not only healthcare clinics). Sections within each chapter will introduce core ethnographic concepts and techniques and consider how to apply them in pragmatic research, complete with lessons learned and examples. To complement our chapters, our colleagues provide case studies, describing pragmatic ethnographic research in healthcare settings. Cases illustrate both the "how-to" and the value of ethnographic approaches. Throughout the book, we refer to case study authors and ourselves by first names after the first mention as a way to include readers in our community of pragmatic ethnographers. We refer to the work of other scholars in the field using last names following academic citation practices.

In Chapter 2, we explore ways to determine when ethnography is a good methodological fit, including research questions that are well-suited for ethnography and sampling and site selection approaches that are a good fit for pragmatic healthcare ethnography. Key points are illustrated via a case study of using ethnographic approaches in pharmacy research. Chapter 3 offers extensive guidance about using ethnographic methods in healthcare environments. (Those who are less familiar with qualitative methods may benefit from reading this chapter before Chapter 2.) Two case studies exemplify participatory ethnographic methods that feature lived experiences and actionable results. In Chapter 4, we explore analytic approaches in pragmatic healthcare ethnography, first considering analytic goals and needs and then briefly describing analytic tools that we have found helpful in our ethnographic work. Analytic rigor is discussed and then illustrated via a case study that describes the analysis of ethnographic data as a participatory endeavor. Chapter 5 explores moving from analysis to write-up of ethnographic findings, covering a variety of potential products. A case study highlights a multifaceted dissemination strategy involving formats tailored to different audiences. In Chapter 6, we examine new opportunities in pragmatic healthcare ethnography, including theoretical and methodological innovations as well as trends in learning health system conceptualizations that speak to the relevance and importance of ethnography in health and health care.

Case 1

Thinking (and acting) ethnographically in VA healthcare research

Heather Schacht Reisinger

Statement 1: Ethnography is an epistemology.

Statement 2: Ethnography is historically and theoretically rooted in the discipline of anthropology.

The interconnection between these two statements underlies this case study on using ethnography as a tool for creating change. Starting here forces a step back to not just talking about the nuts and bolts of the content or what makes up ethnography as a methodology—going to the site, conducting interviews, observation, and so on—but to how ethnographers *act as ethnographers*. The case study attempts to do all of the above in its description of an ethnographic use case.

First, the case demonstrates how ethnography as an epistemology defines the way ethnographers sit among the people we hope to understand. This also requires time away from the people and their space to have time to reflect and piece things together. And then returning to sit among them again with a renewed understanding to test and reexamine what we think we have learned. All of this is about working with participants as partners in building a shared, or translatable, picture of what they taught the ethnographers.

Second, the epistemology of ethnography is rooted in its home discipline of anthropology—the discipline with the longest history of engaging this methodology—and three of its central characteristics: the emic perspective, cultural relativity, and holism (see Box 1.1). These tenets can be seen as both goals and values. The emic perspective is an insider's perspective. The goal of the ethnographer is to ask people to explain the topic of interest from their own way of understanding and seeing the issue. The only way to come close to comprehending an emic perspective is for an ethnographer to pay attention to how she is sitting with people and value what they say and do and their explanations of why. These actions are based on cultural relativity—an assumption that all cultural values must be understood within their own cultural context and not judged according to external standards, requiring an act of nonjudgment on the part of ethnographers. Finally, as Alison, Gemmae, and Erin note, ethnographers strive for a holistic perspective, a full understanding of the question of study and its potential answers. Ethnographers value the goal of a full and comprehensive understanding, even while acknowledging it may not be possible to achieve; this value encourages ongoing respect for participants, who emerge as critical teachers in the research process.

This case seeks to be an example of ethnography as epistemology—what it looks like to think, be, sit, act, listen, step back, and examine with these three anthropologically-rooted characteristics of the emic perspective, cultural relativism, and holism.

Ethnography as a tool for change

Like most of the cases in this book, this case is situated in the VA. One of the challenges VA faces is effectively treating veterans with post-traumatic stress disorder (PTSD). The cumulative research evidence indicates that the so-called "exposure therapies" are among the most effective for treating PTSD (Eftekhari et al. 2013). These therapies require special training for one person, a therapist, to help guide another person, in this case a veteran patient, through the treatment protocol. The problem is that there is often a mismatch between where those specially trained therapists are and the veterans in need of treatment (Brooks et al. 2012; Dufort et al. 2021; Rosen et al. 2019).

In part, this mismatch occurs because the VA must provide care for veterans across the United States and its territories. To provide this care, VA has a network of community-based outpatient clinics that offer primary care and mental health services. These outpatient clinics are affiliated with a main VA medical center and extend their reach so veterans can access care closer to home if they do not live near a medical center. Many of the outpatient clinics are in rural communities and serve rural veterans. While these clinics are required to have mental health services available, many do not have therapists specifically trained in exposure therapy protocols, such as prolonged exposure (PE) therapy or cognitive processing therapy (CPT). Research has shown that rural veterans with PTSD treated at these clinics experience little to no improvement in their symptoms over time (Fortney et al. 2015). Research also demonstrates that exposure therapies are not being provided in these outpatient clinic settings (Grubbs et al. 2017), and that—even when veterans are able to access exposure therapies—they may struggle to remain engaged with these therapies (Kehle-Forbes et al. 2016).

Based on this research, Dr. John Fortney, a VA health services researcher, developed an intervention called Telemedicine Outreach for PTSD (TOP). TOP consists of a care manager, a telepsychologist, and a telepsychiatrist at the VAMC providing specialty mental health care to veterans in these outpatient clinics. The care manager is critical to TOP and serves many roles in support of the veteran. First, the care manager maintains and reviews a casefinder, which is a list of veterans diagnosed with PTSD but not receiving specialty mental health services. The care manager reaches out to the veterans on the casefinder and conducts motivational interviewing to encourage the veteran to enroll in exposure therapy. Once enrolled in therapy, the care manager continues to reach out to the veterans to help ensure they remain engaged—and compliant—with treatment. Compliance to the exposure therapies for PTSD (PE and CPT) includes weekly attendance and homework assignments. The care manager also checks in with the veteran to discuss any barriers they are facing and brainstorm solutions to help facilitate their success in treatment.

After developing this program, Dr. Fortney conducted a randomized controlled trial at 11 community-based outpatient clinics in four states (Fortney et al. 2015). The original research team found 54.9% of veterans randomized to TOP initiated an evidence-based psychotherapy compared to 12.1% of veterans in usual care. In addition, 27.1% of veterans randomized to TOP completed ≥8 sessions of the evidence-based psychotherapy compared to 5.3% of veterans in usual care. Most importantly, veterans in TOP had significantly larger reductions in PTSD symptom severity at 6- and 12-month follow-ups.

Based on these findings, Dr. Fortney received funding from the VA Quality Enhancement Research Initiative (QUERI), VA's national program funding implementation efforts, to conduct a trial of standardized and enhanced implementation strategies. Using a stepped-wedge design (Brown and Lilford 2006), all sites implemented TOP based on a standard implementation strategy, which involved the distribution of an intervention manual and monthly calls among site leads. If sites failed the benchmark (i.e., <20% veterans on the casefinder enrolled in an evidence-based psychotherapy for PTSD), they were then randomly assigned to receive an enhanced implementation strategy or continue as usual. The enhanced implementation strategy involved external facilitation informed by an ethnographic Rapid Assessment Process (RAP).

RAP is defined as "intensive, team-based qualitative inquiry using triangulation, iterative analysis and additional data collection to quickly develop a preliminary understanding of a situation from the insider's perspective" (Beebe 2001: xv). This methodology has had several names over the years, including rapid rural appraisal, rapid assessment process/procedures/protocol, and rapid qualitative inquiry. RAP and similar methods originated when anthropologists were hired in the 1960s and 1970s to work for international development agencies to answer questions such as: When we take an effective intervention from one country and move it to another country, why does it not have the same effect? And what do we need to change to make it effective again? (Reisinger et al. 2021).

The key components of RAP include:

- a focused question with focused analysis;
- team-based approach (multi-disciplinary, preferably a team that includes individuals working in the topical/clinical area);
- going to the location/setting;
- methods traditionally associated with ethnography (direct observation, open-ended interviews and focus groups, surveys, organizational and archival documents, mapping sites); and
- an ethnographic epistemology, that is, leaning into an insider perspective, withholding judgment, and striving for comprehensive, holistic understanding.

To use RAP to inform the external facilitation team, two ethnographers (Heather and Dr. Jane Moeckli) conducted three site visits to VA medical centers and their affiliated community-based outpatient clinics who failed to reach the 20% benchmark. They interviewed care managers, site project leads, telepsychologists, telepsychiatrists, other mental health providers, outpatient clinic providers, and leadership at each of the sites. They conducted all of the interviews in person, often driving several hours between the main medical center and outpatient clinic. While at each site, they also asked the staff to give them a tour to see where veterans would go to meet with the tele-providers and to observe the process for completing therapy sessions via telehealth. They recorded the interviews and took extensive notes on their observations. They then debriefed, often during the long car rides, and began to sketch out maps of the clinical workflow of each site. These clinical workflow maps included both the clinical care process and potential implementation barriers they had heard during their interviews. These sketches became a map of their ethnographic visit and, more importantly, represented how veterans and tele-therapists connected for the delivery of PTSD treatment.

To inform external facilitation, the ethnographers formalized the clinical workflow maps in Visio software, reviewed the workflows with the full external facilitation team (Dr. Fortney and JP Smith, a veteran who had successfully completed TOP), and made clarifying revisions in response to Dr. Fortney's and JP's questions as the members of the external facilitation team who did not participate in the site visits. As the external facilitation team, Dr. Fortney, JP, Dr. Moeckli, and Heather also came up with a plan for discussing the workflow with the medical center team where the site visit took place. Once the workflow and plan were finalized, they set up external facilitation visits (either in-person or virtually) with medical center staff.

Something unexpected happened when the external facilitation team shared the clinical workflows with the medical center teams. The teams frequently said something like, "This is the first time we have seen our whole practice on one page." Then rich conversations occurred around why things were set up the way they were and what things could be changed to address barriers to the implementation of TOP. During those conversations, the medical center and external facilitation teams redesigned the workflow maps, which provided those involved in the conversations a shared point of focus.

Next in the process, the external facilitation team revised the visual representation of the workflow in Visio and shared it back out with the medical center team. Sometimes additional revisions needed to take place, but at some point each team agreed on a workflow and began to implement the newly designed flow.

Ethnographic epistemology in RAP

This case represented an opportunity to use ethnography as a tool for change—as an implementation strategy, to use the nomenclature of the field of implementation science (Powell et al. 2015; Waltz et al. 2015). Central to ethnography being a tool of change in this case is its epistemology. First, the ethnographers practiced *cultural relativism* in how they showed up in clinics, listened to the varying perspectives, and observed the practices (see Box 1.3). The collecting of data was done without judgment. Second, the case represented striving for holism. The clinical workflow maps were an attempt to put the "whole practice" on one page. This became a tool for change because it provided a *holistic* picture that not everyone had seen, imagined, or shared before. Finally, it also represented an *emic perspective* in an interesting way. The ethnographers were responsible for taking all of the emic perspectives—from care managers to mental health providers at outpatient clinics to telepsychologists—and drawing a picture of how they fit together. Each person in the meeting saw themself in the picture, but likely in a different way because they had to understand their perspective in relation to another emic perspective that they may not have been aware of previously. As they heard and saw their team members' emic perspectives in a holistic picture, they each had to adjust their own to a new perspective that could be represented on the same page as their colleagues' perspectives.

Together these actions went beyond the methods of interviewing, taking fieldnotes, and mapping a site. They were driven by an epistemology in which the way the ethnographers acted with the people they were talking with and observing in the space into

Box 1.3 Reflecting on trust and cultural relativism in an ongoing ethnography

One day I was on a site visit and a colleague who was not trained in ethnography asked if he could join me during my interviews. Over the course of the day, I interviewed people who were: 1) recipients of the intervention, some of whom were very disgruntled with the intervention, and 2) delivers of the intervention, some of whom were very frustrated with the lack of engagement of the recipients. I sat with them individually in their private spaces from a stance of cultural relativism and asked them to elaborate on each of their perspectives, empathized with where they were coming from, and sought to understand the intervention from their own, emic perspective. As we got done for the day, we were walking out to the car and my colleague said to me, "I'm never going to trust a thing you say to me again" and laughed. "I watched you go from one person to another with opposing opinions and act as if you believe both." I laughed and quickly said, "How else am I supposed to get a full (i.e., holistic) understanding of [the intervention] and how it is working in practice?" However, that moment still sits with me. I highly value trust. When my colleague said, "I will never trust a thing you say again," my stomach dropped because his comment shook me up. I never want to lose the trust of my colleague and I also never want to lose the trust of any of the people who take the time to sit with me.

I argue this space is the epistemology of ethnography—and that it is essential for doing ethnography well.

(Heather Schact Reisinger)

which they were invited was critical. They also acted by stepping away, reflecting, and returning to share, relearn, and connect. Ethnography is about content, methods, and a way of acting with people in their space as they explain what they value—with a holistic understanding being the goal.

References

Ajjawi, Rola, Joanne Hilder, Christy Noble, Andrew Teodorczuk, and Stephen Billett. 2020. "Using Video-reflexive Ethnography to Understand Complexity and Change Practice." *Medical Education* 54 (10): 908–14. https://doi.org/10.1111/medu.14156.

Beebe, James. 2001. *Rapid Assessment Process: An Introduction.* Walnut Creek, CA: AltaMira Press.

Bernard, H. Russell. 2018. *Research Methods in Anthropology: Qualitative and Quantitative Approaches*, 6th ed. Lanham, Boulder, New York, London: Rowman & Littlefield.

Bikker, Annemieke P., H. Helen Atherton, Brant, Tania Porqueddu, John L. Campbell, Andy Gibson, Brian McKinstry, Chris Salisbury, and Sue Ziebland. 2017. "Conducting a Team-Based Multi-Sited Focused Ethnography in Primary Care." *BMC Medical Research Methodology* 17 (1): 139. https://doi.org/10.1186/s12874-017-0422-5.

Black, Georgia B., Sandra Van Os, Samantha Machen, and Naomi J. Fulop. 2021. "Ethnographic Research as an Evolving Method for Supporting Healthcare Improvement Skills: A Scoping Review." *BMC Medical Research Methodology* 21 (1): 274. https://doi.org/10.1186/s12874-021-01466-9.

Brooks, Elizabeth, Douglas K. Novins, Deborah Thomas, Luohua Jiang, Herbert T. Nagamoto, Nancy Dailey, Byron Bair, and Jay H. Shore. 2012. "Personal Characteristics Affecting Veterans' Use of Services for Posttraumatic Stress Disorder." *Psychiatric Services* 63 (9): 862–67. https://doi.org/10.1176/appi.ps.201100444.

Brown, Celia A., and Richard J. Lilford. 2006. "The Stepped Wedge Trial Design: A Systematic Review." *BMC Medical Research Methodology* 6 (1): 54. https://doi.org/10.1186/1471-2288-6-54.

Cubellis, Lauren, Christine Schmid, and Sebastian Von Peter. 2021. "Ethnography in Health Services Research: Oscillation between Theory and Practice." *Qualitative Health Research* 31 (11): 2029–40. https://doi.org/10.1177/10497323211022312.

Davis, Christine S., and Deborah C. Breede. 2015. "Holistic Ethnography: Embodiment, Emotion, Contemplation, and Dialogue in Ethnographic Fieldwork." *Journal of Contemplative Ethnography* 2 (1): Article 5. https://digscholarship.unco.edu/joci/vol2/iss1/5.

Dixon-Woods, Mary 2003. "What Can Ethnography Do for Quality and Safety in Health Care?" *Quality and Safety in Health Care* 12 (5): 326–27. https://doi.org/10.1136/qhc.12.5.326.

Dufort, Vincent M., Nancy Bernardy, Shira Maguen, Jessica E. Hoyt, Eric R. Litt, Olga V. Patterson, Christine E. Leonard, and Brian Shiner. 2021. "Geographic Variation in Initiation of Evidence-Based Psychotherapy among Veterans With PTSD." *Military Medicine* 186 (9–10): e858–66. https://doi.org/10.1093/milmed/usaa389.

Eftekhari, Afsoon, Josef I. Ruzek, Jill J. Crowley, Craig S. Rosen, Mark A. Greenbaum, and Bradley E Karlin. 2013. "Effectiveness of National Implementation of Prolonged Exposure Therapy in Veterans Affairs Care." *JAMA Psychiatry* 70 (9): 949–55.

Finley, Erin P. 2011. *Fields of Combat: Understanding PTSD among Veterans of Iraq and Afghanistan*. Ithaca, NY: Cornell University Press.

Finley, Erin P., Svea Closser, Malabika Sarker, and Alison B. Hamilton. 2023. "Editorial: The Theory and Pragmatics of Power and Relationships in Implementation." *Frontiers in Health Services* 3: 1168559. https://doi.org/10.3389/frhs.2023.1168559.

Fix, Gemmae M., Justeen K. Hyde, Rendelle E. Bolton, Victoria A. Parker, Kelly Dvorin, Juliet Wu, and Avy A. Skolnik, et al. 2018. "The Moral Discourse of HIV Providers within Their Organizational Context: An Ethnographic Case Study." *Patient Education and Counseling* 101 (12): 2226–32. https://doi.org/10.1016/j.pec.2018.08.018.

Fix, Gemmae M., Bo Kim, Mollie A. Ruben, and Megan B. McCullough. 2022. "Direct Observation Methods: A Practical Guide for Health Researchers." *PEC Innovation* 1: 100036. https://doi.org/10.1016/j.pecinn.2022.100036.

Fortney, John C., Jeffrey M. Pyne, Timothy A. Kimbrell, Teresa J. Hudson, Dean E. Robinson, Ronald Schneider, William M. Moore, Paul J. Custer, Kathleen M. Grubbs, and Paula P. Schnurr. 2015. "Telemedicine-Based Collaborative Care for Posttraumatic Stress Disorder: A Randomized Clinical Trial." *JAMA Psychiatry* 72 (1): 58–67. https://doi.org/10.1001/jamapsychiatry.2014.1575.

Gertner, Alex K., Joshua Franklin, Isabel Roth, Gracelyn H. Cruden, Amber D. Haley, Erin P. Finley, Alison B. Hamilton, Lawrence A. Palinkas, and Byron J. Powell. 2021. "A Scoping Review of the Use of Ethnographic Approaches in Implementation Research and Recommendations for Reporting." *Implementation Research and Practice* 2: 263348952199274. https://doi.org/10.1177/2633489521992743.

Glasgow, Russell E. 2013. "What Does It Mean to Be Pragmatic? Pragmatic Methods, Measures, and Models to Facilitate Research Translation." *Health Education & Behavior* 40 (3): 257–65. https://doi.org/10.1177/1090198113486805.

Grubbs, Kathleen M., John C. Fortney, Tim Kimbrell, Jeffrey M. Pyne, Teresa Hudson, Dean Robinson, William Mark Moore, Paul Custer, Ronald Schneider, and Paula P. Schnurr. 2017. "Usual Care for Rural Veterans with Posttraumatic Stress Disorder." *The Journal of Rural Health* 33 (3): 290–96. https://doi.org/10.1111/jrh.12230.

Hamilton, Alison. 2012. "The Vital Conjuncture of Methamphetamine-involved Pregnancy: Objective Risks and Subjective Realities." In *Risk, Reproduction, and Narratives of Experience*, 59–77. Lauren Fordyce & Aminata Maraesa, Editors. Nashville, TN: Vanderbilt University Press.

Hinder, Susan, and Trisha Greenhalgh. 2012. "'This Does My Head In'. Ethnographic Study of Self-Management by People with Diabetes." *BMC Health Services Research* 12 (1): 83. https://doi.org/10.1186/1472-6963-12-83.

Kehle-Forbes, Shannon M., Laura A. Meis, Michele R. Spoont, and Melissa A. Polusny. 2016. "Treatment Initiation and Dropout from Prolonged Exposure and Cognitive Processing Therapy in a VA Outpatient Clinic." *Psychological Trauma: Theory, Research, Practice, and Policy* 8 (1): 107–14. https://doi.org/10.1037/tra0000065.

Knauft, Bruce. 1996. "Chapter 7: Gender, Ethnography, and Critical Query." In *Genealogies for the Present in Cultural Anthropology*, 219–47. New York: Routledge.

Morgan-Trimmer, Sarah, and Fiona Wood. 2016. "Ethnographic Methods for Process Evaluations of Complex Health Behaviour Interventions." *Trials* 17 (1): 232. https://doi.org/10.1186/s13063-016-1340-2.

Neuwirth, Esther B., Jim Bellows, Ana H. Jackson, and Patricia M. Price. 2012. "How Kaiser Permanente Uses Video Ethnography of Patients for Quality Improvement, Such As in Shaping Better Care Transitions." *Health Affairs* 31 (6): 1244–50. https://doi.org/10.1377/hlthaff.2012.0134.

Palinkas, Lawrence A., and Douglas Zatzick. 2019. "Rapid Assessment Procedure Informed Clinical Ethnography (RAPICE) in Pragmatic Clinical Trials of Mental Health Services Implementation: Methods and Applied Case Study." *Administration and Policy in Mental Health and Mental Health Services Research* 46 (2): 255–70. https://doi.org/10.1007/s10488-018-0909-3.

Powell, Byron J., Thomas J. Waltz, Matthew J. Chinman, Laura J. Damschroder, Jeffrey L. Smith, Monica M. Matthieu, Enola K. Proctor, and JoAnn E. Kirchner. 2015. "A Refined Compilation of Implementation Strategies: Results from the Expert Recommendations for Implementing Change (ERIC) Project." *Implementation Science* 10 (1): 21. https://doi.org/10.1186/s13012-015-0209-1.

Reisinger, Heather Schacht, John Fortney, and Greg Reger. 2021. "Rapid Ethnographic Assessment in Clinical Settings." In *Paths to the Future of Higher Education*, 117–34. Brian L. Foster, Steven W. Graham, and Joe F. Donaldson, Editors. Charlotte, NC: Information Age.

Rosen, Craig S., Nancy C. Bernardy, Kathleen M. Chard, Barbara Clothier, Joan M. Cook, Jill Crowley, and Afsoon Eftekhari, et al. 2019. "Which Patients Initiate Cognitive Processing Therapy and Prolonged Exposure in Department of Veterans Affairs PTSD Clinics?" *Journal of Anxiety Disorders* 62: 53–60. https://doi.org/10.1016/j.janxdis.2018.11.003.

Savage, Jan. 2006. "Ethnographic Evidence: The Value of Applied Ethnography in Healthcare." *Journal of Research in Nursing* 11 (5): 383–93. https://doi.org/10.1177/1744987106068297.

Snell-Rood, Claire, Elise Trott Jaramillo, Alison B. Hamilton, Sarah E. Raskin, Francesca M. Nicosia, and Cathleen Willging. 2021. "Advancing Health Equity through a Theoretically Critical Implementation Science." *Translational Behavioral Medicine* 11 (8): 1617–25. https://doi.org/10.1093/tbm/ibab008.

Trundle, Catherine, and Tarryn Phillips. 2023. "Defining Focused Ethnography: Disciplinary Boundary-Work and the Imagined Divisions between 'Focused' and 'Traditional' Ethnography in Health Research – A Critical Review." *Social Science & Medicine* 332: 116108. https://doi.org/10.1016/j.socscimed.2023.116108.

Vindrola-Padros, Cecilia, and Bruno Vindrola-Padros. 2018. "Quick and Dirty? A Systematic Review of the Use of Rapid Ethnographies in Healthcare Organisation and Delivery." *BMJ Quality and Safety* 27 (4): 321–30. https://doi.org/10.1136/bmjqs-2017-007226.

Waltz, Thomas J., Byron J. Powell, Monica M. Matthieu, Laura J. Damschroder, Matthew J. Chinman, Jeffrey L. Smith, Enola K. Proctor, and JoAnn E. Kirchner. 2015. "Use of Concept Mapping to Characterize Relationships Among Implementation Strategies and Assess Their Feasibility and Importance: Results from the Expert Recommendations for Implementing Change (ERIC) Study." *Implementation Science* 10 (1): 109. https://doi.org/10.1186/s13012-015-0295-0.

CHAPTER 2

Designing ethnography for healthcare research

Introduction

When we have a research question that may be best addressed using an ethnographic study design, where do we begin? For most ethnographic studies, the first step is to develop the set of methods (e.g., interviews and observation) that will be integrated to answer the research questions, with careful consideration of feasibility and suitability. In this chapter, we outline core principles for designing pragmatic ethnography to address focused topics in healthcare settings (i.e., any settings where health occurs or health care happens). We first describe what types of research questions are a good fit for ethnographic methods, then provide a brief overview of common methods and their key functions, before considering how to select and assemble a cohesive set of methods for a specific study, weighing critical issues in sampling, and diving into the nitty-gritty of access and approvals for ethnographic studies. (We will go into more detail on the specifics of ethnographic data collection in Chapter 3.)

When are ethnographic methods a good fit for healthcare research?

In considering this question, it can help to begin with an example. In one of Gemmae's early studies, she sought to address the research question of how patients' social environments influenced recovery from open-heart surgery (Fix and Bokhour 2012). Her study was informed by the biocultural model of health (McElroy and Townsend 2014), which conceptualizes health as occurring at the intersection of the biotic (i.e., biologic environment), abiotic (i.e., physical environment), and socio-cultural environments. She drew upon this holistic model in developing her study design: data collection included assessments of clinical, biological data (blood pressure, weight), the physical environment (patients were interviewed and observed both in the hospital and in their homes), and the socio-cultural environment (with attention in both the interviews and observations of the people in the patients' lives). The resulting ethnographic study combined multiple methods, included both patients and providers, and accounted for clinical,

DOI: 10.4324/9781003390657-2

quantitative as well as qualitative data. As a result, Gemmae was able to illuminate how widely divergent patient and provider perspectives were on what "recovery" meant. For example, one provider stated that a patient had recovered when they went home from the hospital, indicating their focus on the surgery and the hospital setting. In contrast, patients situated their recovery in the context of their households. It was in their homes and with their families that they made decisions about meals and activities, not solely based on their own health needs.

As in this example, ethnographic approaches are ideal for understanding context-specific phenomena, insiders' perspectives, and complex interactions between individuals, groups, and/or structural factors such as local and broader environments, structures, or policies (Gertner et al. 2021). Often, pragmatic healthcare ethnography begins with a health-related problem, such as: Why are patients not taking their medication? Why aren't doctors adopting an evidence-based treatment that could improve care for their patients? Why is there so much variation in clinical outcomes across hospitals in a healthcare system? But where qualitative research methods like interviewing can work independently to answer relatively narrow questions—for example, how do patients feel about recovery from open-heart surgery—ethnographic approaches go a step further. Ethnographic methods can place those feelings in the context of the broader environment, illuminating, for example, why providers may not fully appreciate how difficult it can be to recover at home, why some patients face an easier recovery than others, or how insurance policies or the broader healthcare system may shape access to post-surgery supports and resources, like access to physical therapy. Integrating the results of diverse methods can allow for seeing patterns across multiple perspectives and types of data. Said another way, ethnography generates more than the sum of its methods.

However, ethnography is not always a good fit for a particular research question or opportunity, because of issues related to suitability, accessibility, or feasibility (see Table 2.1). Researchers should first consider whether an ethnographic approach is suitable to answer the research question(s). For example, ethnography would be

Table 2.1 Questions to consider when deciding whether ethnography is appropriate for a given study

Issue	*Questions to consider*
Suitability to the research question	■ Will an ethnographic study design provide findings to answer the research question(s)? ■ Is a multi-method ethnographic study required, or would a single-method qualitative research design (e.g., using interviews) suffice?
Accessibility	■ Is the population, event, or behavior, taboo, hidden, or otherwise inaccessible? ■ Will we be able to gain physical or virtual access to the setting?
Frequency	■ Is the event or behavior frequent enough to capture?
Approvals	■ Do we have time for institutional ethical review? ■ Do we have permission from key oversight bodies? ■ Is permission needed from other key parties, such as the clinical lead, facility lead, or other national regulatory bodies?

unlikely to provide appropriate data to statistically demonstrate cause and effect or to deliver generalizable findings across a broad range of contexts. Moreover, some research questions might be answerable using individual interviews or focus groups and not require a full multi-method approach. Accessibility is a key issue. Ethnography may not be a good fit when access to settings, behaviors, events, and/or groups of people is not available or appropriate. For example, a researcher might want to understand the experiences of children with autism or adults with Alzheimer's disease in the emergency department setting. While these would be interesting topics, they both could result in a lot of time spent in the emergency department, with few people meeting study inclusion criteria, and finding ethical strategies for informed consent among participants could pose additional challenges. Accessibility, frequency, and approvals are among the most common reasons an ethnographic study design may not be feasible.

To summarize, then, ethnographic approaches can be invaluable when there is a health-related problem that cannot be explained with existing knowledge, in understanding the context in which health care is occurring, and in understanding change over time, whether planned (e.g., when implementing a new intervention) or unplanned (e.g., responding to increasing rates of provider burnout). An ethnographic design can also be a good fit for research questions that require information about what people are doing in their everyday settings, interactions, and relationships. The case studies featured throughout this book illustrate a wide range of research questions explored using an ethnographic approach (see Box 2.1). Reviewing these, we can notice that they share core features of effective research questions in pragmatic healthcare ethnography: they are primarily "how" and "what" questions; they aim to understand the interaction *between* phenomena (e.g., between healthcare efforts and outcomes); they state the population of interest; and they focus on a particular health condition (e.g., PTSD) or healthcare setting/context where the problem is happening (in this case, all within VA healthcare).

Box 2.1 Sample research questions explored in ethnographic case studies in this book

- How do local outpatient clinic workflows inhibit or facilitate veterans' enrollment in evidence-based psychotherapies for PTSD? (Case 1: Heather Reisinger)
- How do clinical pharmacy practitioners deliver substance use disorder care in the context of interprofessional clinical teams? (Case 2: Megan McCullough)
- What are the benefits of time in nature for veterans, and how might veteran-centered eco-therapeutic opportunities be created? (Case 3a: Anais Tuepker)
- How can healthcare providers, public health researchers, and concerned community members work together to promote secure firearm storage messaging and practices to prevent suicide by firearm? (Case 3b: Gala True)
- What roles do clerical staff play in primary care settings, and how do these roles impact patient experiences of care? (Case 4: Sarah Ono)
- How do sites implementing a new patient-centered Whole Health initiative go about implementation, and what factors affect their progress? (Case 5: Justeen Hyde)

Methods: The building blocks of an ethnographic study design

Once an initial research question has been identified, we can begin thinking about the specific methods needed to address the research question. The research question can be thought of as the North Star that guides key study features like methods, setting, and population. Throughout this book, we emphasize the need for "methodological coherence," with the research question(s) guiding study design and method selection, data collection, data analysis, and later synthesis and write up or other sharing of findings (Morse et al. 2002). As the foundation for ensuring this coherence, selecting complementary methods to be layered and integrated into ethnographic findings is essential. The methods provide the building blocks of the study design. Methods commonly used in healthcare ethnography include individual and focus group interviews, observation, document review, surveys, and analysis of administrative data (e.g., from an electronic health record). Although we discuss many of these methods in detail in Chapter 3, it is useful to offer a brief overview of them here (see Table 2.2), so we can begin to think about how they can be assembled to meet the needs of ethnographic studies. *Bringing together an integrated set of methods that is carefully tailored to the research question(s) is a hallmark of good ethnographic study design.*

Individual interviews are among the most commonly used qualitative research methods, not least because they are a flexible tool for developing an understanding of individual perspectives and experiences. They are well-suited to a variety of topics, including those that may be more sensitive or taboo, and allow for gathering person-centered

Table 2.2 A brief overview of common methods in ethnographic studies

Method	*Best use*	*Benefits*	*Challenges*
Individual interviews	■ Understand perspectives and experiences	■ Allow for person-centered narrative ■ Better for sensitive or taboo topics	■ Participant logistics (identification, recruitment, scheduling, conducting)
Focus groups	■ Foster discussion about a phenomenon	■ Allow for generative brainstorming ■ Constrain data collection to a single event	■ Unequal contributions ■ Less predictable ■ Considerable work identifying a time that works for all
Observation	■ Learn what people are doing and how they interact ■ Identify previously unrecognized behaviors or phenomena	■ Provide an opportunity to observe and document normative practice ■ Illuminate tacit behaviors	■ Getting access ■ Hard to observe subtle or taboo behaviors
Document/archival review	■ Investigate material evidence of a phenomenon ■ Provide historical context	■ Existing data ■ May provide "official"/approved narratives	■ Getting access ■ Limited to what the author recorded

narratives. Their challenges include identifying and recruiting potential participants, scheduling interviews, and finding a safe, private, and comfortable place or format (i.e., video or phone), to conduct them.

Focus groups, by contrast, are ideal for opening dialogue about a phenomenon in order to develop a nuanced understanding of a shared experience (e.g., a clinical workflow, caregiver experiences of post-discharge care for a family member, a healthcare condition), and to elicit areas of agreement and disagreement. They can allow for generative brainstorming (e.g., hashing out ideas for a new intervention or identifying potential pitfalls of an upcoming initiative) and can be efficient for gathering multiple perspectives in a short period of time. Their limitations are inherent to the group format, which may result in some participants talking and getting more "air time" than others. They can be unpredictable and difficult to manage in a way that is both comfortable for everyone and generative of relevant information, particularly where the personalities and group dynamics are unknown to the researcher. Moreover, they can be difficult to schedule, as they require finding a single time that works well for all the participants.

Observation, although not required for a study to be considered "ethnographic," is a hallmark method for coming to understand what people are doing and how they interact, and can be invaluable for understanding normative practice. Particularly when combined with interviewing or focus groups, observation can provide a lens onto the difference between what people say (report, believe) and what they actually *do* in day-to-day practice, thus offering insight into phenomena that may otherwise go unreported or unnoticed. However, getting access to the spaces where relevant events are occurring may be difficult, particularly if privacy or protected information is a concern, which is often the case in healthcare environments (we'll say more about this later on). Moreover, it can be hard to observe taboo behaviors, such as those related to sexual behavior or substance use, or even just behaviors considered "private."

Finally, *document or other archival review* means reviewing existing data sources to understand how events or policies are documented or reported, particularly in the "official" record. They can provide historical context for how a phenomenon emerged or the rationale behind it. In health care, perhaps the most common example of using this method would be a chart review of providers' notes about a group of patients or specific health condition; for example, reviewing how providers describe symptoms of dementia among new patients and whether those descriptions vary by the ethnicity of the provider or patient. Meeting agendas or minutes can also provide systematic, structured information.

Each of these methods (as well as many more!) can offer a unique lens onto a specific research problem and question, with the combination into a multi-method approach providing holistic perspective. In the ethnographic example that opened this chapter, Gemmae's research question examined the relationship between patients' socio-cultural environment and their post-surgical health. To build a deep, multifaceted understanding, Gemmae wanted to observe and speak with a variety of people who could provide insight on what factors affected patients' recovery. She therefore selected interviews as one focal method, conducted with both patients who had open-heart surgery and their surgical team. She also collected clinical data relevant to patients' cardiac health, like their weight and blood pressure, and survey data about their health-related quality of

Table 2.3 Example patient data collection plan (Fix 2008)

Research phase	*Time for patient*	*Data collection*
I. Recruitment	Pre-surgery Clinic appointment	Brief interview Medical records Anthropometrics Health survey
Surgery	*No patient contact* 0 weeks	Medical record (surgery-related information such as date, procedure, and any peri-surgical complications)
II. Phone call	7 weeks	Brief interview Health survey
III. Household assessment	15 weeks	In-home interview, observation Anthropometrics (i.e., weight and blood pressure) Health survey
IV. Follow-up phone call	20 weeks	Brief interview Medical records Health survey

life. Table 2.3 provides a summary of data collected from patients as part of the study, and Table 2.4 indicates the sample and sample sizes.

In addition to interviews and the collection of clinical data, Gemmae elected to include observation in her study. She conducted in-home visits with patients to observe their day-to-day living and local environment. She was able to observe key events for two patients in the hospital: the day of surgery and the in-hospital recovery period. She also spent a day following an anesthesiology fellow who was part of the surgical team and a day following the physician's assistant, who worked closely with patients as they recovered in the hospital. And finally, Gemmae conducted general observations of the cardiothoracic service's clinic, team meetings, and meetings with cardiology. When integrated, these multiple perspectives (patient, provider; hospital, home) and sources of data (medical record, survey, interviews, and observations) allowed for a holistic description of the recovery experience while also providing insight into how it might be improved.

Planning an ethnographic study

When developing an ethnographic study, it can be helpful to ask a series of questions (see Table 2.5), often starting with why, what, how, who, when, and where. "Why" and "what" questions include thinking about what methods can best help to answer

Table 2.4 Example of study participants (Fix 2008)

Component	*Participants*	*Total N (41)*
Surgical recovery	Patients	37
In-hospital follows	Clinicians	2
	Surgical patients	2

Table 2.5 Considerations when planning an ethnographic study design

Why	■ Why use an ethnographic study design? Why is ethnography the preferred approach for the proposed research question(s)?
What	■ What are our end goals? ■ What will we produce? (see Chapter 5) • For what audience(s)?
How	■ How will we conduct the ethnography (see Chapter 3)? • What do we already know going into the field? • What methods will we use and why? • What will be the role of theory? ■ How will we analyze and integrate different data sources (see Chapter 4)?
Who	■ With whom will the ethnography be conducted and why? ■ What is the sampling approach for each method? ■ Who is on the research team?
When	■ When will each method occur and why those timepoints?
Where	■ Where will each method occur?

our research question(s) and initial planning for the end goals and products (which may inform data to be collected). "How" questions start laying out a preliminary plan for what methods will be included, whether and how theory will be used, and how analysis will be approached. "Who" questions consider both who will be part of the ethnographic study team and who the population of interest is, as well as the sampling, locations, and timing/"when" for each method. After the initial methods are selected, thinking through these questions can help to flesh out the broader plan for an ethnographic study design.

Once the overall study design starts to emerge, it becomes easier to begin a second phase of design planning that we like to think of as "getting granular." Later in this chapter, we offer two potential strategies for approaching this, one built around "specific aims," which are the traditional way of structuring a research grant proposal, and one built around a "data summary," which can be a concise way of outlining the goals, methods, and key elements of study design. These approaches offer useful templates for summarizing a research plan.

Table 2.6 illustrates the first approach, which breaks down activities for each specific aim, the intended approach for that aim (including the setting, participants, and methods), and the end goal or desired outcome.

Table 2.6 Study design overview template

Overarching study goal			
	Aim 1	*Aim 2*	*Aim 3*
Specific aim			
Approach (setting, participants, and methods)			
End goal/desired outcome			

Table 2.7 Example study overview

Goal: Co-design an evidence-based plan to provide patient-centered care to people living with HIV			
	Developmental formative evaluation		*Co-design*
	Aim 1	*Aim 2*	*Aim 3*
Specific Aim	Identify predictors of patient-centered "Whole Health" service receipt by patients with HIV.	Examine patients' and providers' perspectives on how to integrate patient-centered "Whole Health" care in HIV specialty care settings.	Co-design an implementation blueprint for integrating patient-centered, "Whole Health" into HIV specialty care, working with veterans w/HIV, providers, and leadership.
Approach	**Quantitative.** Using structured data, a survey, and training data, we will identify patient-, clinic-, & site-level predictors of patient-centered service use in patients w/ HIV at 18 patient-centered hospitals.	**Qualitative.** Through semi-structured, qualitative interviews, explore 40 patients' and 30 HIV providers' ideas about using patient-centered services in HIV care.	**Co-design.** Using our team's co-design framework, we will collaborate w/patient, provider, and leadership stakeholders to develop an implementation blueprint.
Goal	Characterize people with HIV who are using patient-centered services at the 18 hospitals.	Understand patient- and provider-level barriers to patient-centered care for patients with HIV.	Engage end-users to develop a blueprint of implementation strategies tailored to their needs and experiences.

As an example of how this template might look for a completed study, see Table 2.7. Gemmae conducted an ethnographic study with the goal of understanding variation in delivery of patient-centered care services to people living with HIV. She initially developed the table to help think through different key elements of her study plan. Later, the table helped her write the accompanying text of the grant proposal. Gemmae included the table in the grant to help the grant reviewers more easily understand her research plan; it worked—the grant was funded!

Another approach to pulling together details of study design is to develop an overarching data summary (Table 2.8). This data summary format provides a concise study plan on a single page that can serve as a go-to reference in both planning and conducting the study. It includes the specific aims and key research question(s) at the top and then breaks down each method to be included in the study, its participants, the content

Table 2.8 Data summary template

<table>
<tr><td colspan="6">Specific Aims
1.
2.</td></tr>
<tr><td colspan="6">Research Question(s)
1.
2.</td></tr>
<tr><td>Data source/ participants</td><td>Method</td><td>Timing</td><td>Content/variables</td><td>Analytic plan</td><td>Goal/purpose</td></tr>
<tr><td></td><td></td><td></td><td></td><td></td><td></td></tr>
<tr><td></td><td></td><td></td><td></td><td></td><td></td></tr>
<tr><td></td><td></td><td></td><td></td><td></td><td></td></tr>
<tr><td></td><td></td><td></td><td></td><td></td><td></td></tr>
</table>

or variables to be assessed (including key theory constructs, if applicable), the timing of each data collection point, plan for analysis, and intended purpose (i.e., the aim or question addressed). This format provides a prompt to think through many of the most pressing issues in conducting an ethnographic (or other multi-method) study and to assemble a picture of how specific data gathered from multiple vantage points over points in time will cumulatively allow for analysis, synthesis, addressing the research question(s), and developing essential products.

Alison and Erin have used this approach across multiple studies and published a version of this table as part of a resulting manuscript (Huynh et al. 2018). For a completed version summarizing a study of implementing three different evidence-based practices to improve preventive lifestyle and mental health care for women veterans in VA healthcare (Hamilton et al. 2023), see Table 2.9. Even though this latter example illustrates a complex multi-method study with both quantitative and qualitative outcomes of interest (relative to clinical effectiveness and implementation of the different practices), the data summary allows for a comprehensive overview of the study plan. (Several of the methods and analytic strategies described will be discussed in more detail in Chapters 3 and 4.)

Sampling: Site and participant selection

As evident in these examples, one of the most critical steps in getting granular is sampling, by identifying participants and sites. When thinking through possible participants, it can be helpful to consider several questions, such as: who can help explain the issue of interest? Who is involved or impacted? Who is (or is not) receiving the care or services? Who is delivering care or services? Who has relevant oversight or decision-making authority? What other partners should be consulted for input or are needed to complete key activities? Similar questions arise when considering sites: where are the key phenomena occurring? Are some sites struggling more than others with a particular issue, in which case it may be useful to stratify by performance (e.g., high-performing, low-performing) to allow for comparison? How many sites are feasible to include, given the resources of the research team (including timeline and budget)?

Table 2.9 Example data summary for a study of implementing evidence-based practices for women veterans in VA health care (Hamilton et al. 2023)

Specific Aims

1 Using two implementation strategies (Replicating Effective Programs [REP] and Evidence-Based Quality Improvement [EBQI]), support implementation and sustainment of three virtual evidence-based practices (EBPs) focused on preventive lifestyle and mental health care for women veterans across 20 VA facilities (10 REP and 10 EBQI sites).
2 Conduct a mixed methods implementation evaluation using a cluster-randomized hybrid type 3 effectiveness-implementation trial design comparing the effectiveness of REP and EBQI in terms of (a) improved access to and rates of engagement in preventive lifestyle and mental telehealth services (primary outcome) and improved VA performance metrics for telehealth care delivery and related clinical outcomes for women veterans; (b) progression along the Stages of Implementation Completion; (c) adaptation, sensemaking, and experiences of EBP implementation among multilevel stakeholders; and (d) cost and return on investment.
3 Generate implementation "playbooks" for program partners that are scalable and serve as guidance for future implementation of a broader array of evidence-based women's health programs and policies.

Research Question(s)

1 How do sites progress toward—and how many achieve—implementation of EBPs using REP and EBQI implementation strategies?
2 How do the two implementation strategies compare in terms of their impact (improved access to and rates of engagement in relevant services), time to implementation, stakeholder experience, and cost and return on investment?

Data source/ Participants	*Method*	*Timing*	*Content/Variables*	*Analytic plan*	*Goal/Purpose*
VA electronic health record data	Administrative data pulls	Monthly per EBP by site; cumulatively at study close	Number of patients engaged/enrolled in each EBP; engagement in EBP sessions/activities; clinical outcomes and performance measures	Generalized linear models	Understand the effectiveness of EBPs in improving access to and engagement in relevant services and comparison of effects across REP and EBQI sites (Aim 2a)

(Continued)

Table 2.9 (Continued)

Data source/ Participants	*Method*	*Timing*	*Content/Variables*	*Analytic plan*	*Goal/Purpose*
Implementation team members	Periodic reflections*	Monthly with study leads for each EBP and REP and EBQI team members working with sites	Ongoing implementation activities, events, and challenges; opportunities; EBP and/or implementation strategy adaptations; inner and outer setting influences; and planning, processes, and key events.	Rapid qualitative analysis and targeted coding (e.g., of adaptations)**	Understand conditions affecting progress toward implementation (Aim 2b) and experiences of EBP implementation (Aim 2c); inform development of playbook (Aim 3)
	Structured fieldnotes of site implementation meetings ("Call sheets")*	Conducted at implementation team meetings, which may occur monthly, quarterly, or on demand	Meeting date, attendees, topics of discussion (including local challenges and accomplishments), progress on activities, planned next steps, key implementation milestones met (and date)	Analysis as part of Stages of Implementation Completion; rapid qualitative analysis; targeted coding**	Understand conditions affecting progress toward implementation (Aim 2b) and experiences of EBP implementation (Aim 2c); inform assessment of cost and return on investment for each strategy (Aim 2d); inform development of playbook (Aim 3)

(Continued)

Table 2.9 (Continued)

Data source/ Participants	*Method*	*Timing*	*Content/Variables*	*Analytic plan*	*Goal/Purpose*
Regional leadership and site-level participants (frontline staff, providers, and facility leadership)	Semi-structured interviews*	Pre-implementation	Inner and outer context, individual characteristics and experiences, baseline practice, informed by Consolidated Framework for Implementation Research (CFIR: Damschroder et al. 2022)	Rapid qualitative analysis and targeted coding**	Understand conditions affecting progress toward implementation (Aim 2b) and experiences of EBP implementation (Aim 2c)
	Semi-structured interviews*	Post-implementation	Inner and outer context, individual characteristics and experiences, experiences of and reflections on implementation process, informed by CFIR	Rapid qualitative analysis and targeted coding**	Understand conditions affecting progress toward implementation (Aim 2b) and experiences of EBP implementation (Aim 2c)

*See Chapter 3 for additional discussion of these methods.
**See Chapter 4 for additional discussion of these analytic strategies.

Once the most essential participants have been identified, a second critical issue is sample size, possibly of both participants and sites. Sample size in an ethnographic study is about having the right data—and a sufficient amount of the right data—to answer the research question. Traditional ethnographic studies often rely initially on relatively few participants and a strategy of convenience or snowball sampling that allows ethnographers to slowly grow participant networks within their chosen site. We see this approach less commonly in pragmatic healthcare ethnography, where we frequently need to specify our sampling approach early in the process as part of seeking research funding or approvals, as well as to consider practical elements like staffing an appropriately-sized team or budgeting for participant compensation. Moreover, our sample sizes may also be influenced by the nature of the research question. In some types of healthcare research (e.g., health services research), we may aim for larger sample sizes to allow for comparison of findings between groups, for example, comparing experiences of people of different ethnicities in receiving dermatology care. In implementation studies, we often find that sample sizes are limited by the number of people involved in delivery of a specific intervention at a given site, which may be relatively small. And across the spectrum of pragmatic healthcare ethnography, we are nearly always faced with the need to get the work done on a specific timeline, which imposes limitations of its own. We may also have to grapple with how many sites to include in our ethnographic studies, asking key questions such as: how is a site defined (e.g., a specialty clinic within a hospital, an outpatient or residential setting, a hospital, a surgery suite)? How many sites do we need to answer the research question and to accommodate the study design (e.g., if ethnography is part of a larger cluster-randomized trial)? As with participants, determining the sample size of sites is greatly influenced by available resources, with multisite sites typically requiring a large budget.

Whereas it has become common in qualitative research to aim for a sample size of participants that will allow for achieving *saturation*, or the point at which relatively little new information on the topic of interest or theory is emerging from additional participants (Glaser and Strauss 1967), we may need to consider alternative approaches in planning for sampling. Seeking *information power* focuses on ensuring that we are including participants with expertise in the topic of interest, whether via lived experience, training and practice, or routine involvement (Malterud, Siersma, and Guassora 2016). In sampling, we are also looking ahead to our goals for analysis, planning to ensure that we have *conceptual depth* and *sufficiency* of evidence to illustrate key lessons in the data and ensure that those lessons have subtlety and richness of meaning, resonate with existing literature, and stand up to testing (Nelson 2017; Vasileiou et al. 2018). How much data is likely to be needed to understand a phenomenon will also be shaped by the complexity of that phenomenon: simple problems tend to require smaller sample sizes, whereas complex problems may require larger ones to fully understand (Hennink and Kaiser 2022).

A note about "N"

Beware the desire to have a large sample size! Quantitative studies often need to be "powered" to answer a research question because a certain number of participants are needed to run statistical analysis. The number of participants or sites in an ethnographic study is instead driven by the research question, with numbers needed to *sufficiently understand multiple perspectives and phenomena*. Therefore, we consider not only the number of people being interviewed and/or observed but also the number of hours, events, perspectives, and different types of data being brought together. The goal is to have the right amount of data to answer the research question, while also ensuring that planned data collection is feasible and takes into account the need to identify the population, gain access, and engage deeply in interviews, observation, and other data collection and analysis activities.

Getting approval to conduct ethnography in healthcare settings

Once the general study plan begins to emerge (and typically as soon as possible), it is time to begin seeking any necessary approvals to do the work. Seeking permission to access a site or population is part of the ethnographic process. In healthcare settings, official access might come from a supervisor, chief, facility or organizational leader, community leader, or other de facto leadership. Permission may also be needed from informal leadership, such as someone on the clinical staff or a respected community member. These gatekeepers serve an important role in allowing would-be ethnographers entrée into a space. Identifying who key people are should be part of the early planning. This plan should also include how and when to contact them and what the request is. We have found that it is better to over- than under-inform those who might need to know what we plan to do, even if it is not required; this helps to avoid unintended consequences such as a leader being asked why an unfamiliar person is spending time in a particular clinical setting. We have found that leaders appreciate getting a heads up about what is happening in their facility and often want to know what we find!

In Gemmae's doctoral research, the site was one hospital that performed open heart surgery (Fix 2008; Fix and Bokhour 2012). She had a part-time job at the medical school, which gave her access to many of the clinicians at the local hospital, including the Chief of Anesthesiology, who became a key point of contact. He then provided Gemmae entrée to others at the hospital, such as the Chief of Cardio-Thoracic Surgery, the administrative assistant who scheduled patients for surgery, a nurse leader, and staff with the institutional review board (IRB). Having these connections provided Gemmae with a cadre of people she could reach out to when she needed help with specific issues. We share more about building partnerships to support ethnographic research in Chapter 3 and Case Studies 3a and 3b.

Conducting ethnographic work in settings where the researcher already has a role can pose advantages and complexities. There can be tension between being both a clinician who sees patients and a researcher who wants to interview or observe these same patients. If a clinician is conducting research in their own work setting, patients or coworkers may feel obligated to accept an invitation to participate. In an interview, the clinician might have trouble separating their clinical responsibilities from their research curiosities. Research questions differ from clinical ones. If the clinician observes something clinically relevant, how should they respond? These issues need to be thought through when developing the study protocol that outlines each step. One strategy could be to pair clinicians with nonclinical team members or have the clinician serve in an advisory role and not collect research data from patients.

Every research study should be independently assessed by an objective third party, like an IRB or other ethics committee, to ensure it is ethically sound. Getting approval to conduct an ethnographic study in a healthcare setting is not only a legal requirement but also most importantly protects both participants and research team members. The process can be challenging, especially if the reviewing board is unfamiliar with ethnographic methods. Later in this chapter, we provide guidance on how to get ethnographic studies approved by IRBs.

Is it research?

The first question is whether a study is considered research. Research is done to support the broader scientific endeavor to increase generalizable knowledge. It is often published, with publishers requiring documentation of ethical review and approval. Quality improvement (QI), on the other hand, is not typically proposed or designed to increase generalizable knowledge, but rather to improve clinical practice. It is often designed by clinical or operations groups to learn about or address a clinical problem. Both research and QI will typically require review, but QI may receive a determination of nonresearch, depending on institutional regulations. (This determination does not mean that QI work cannot be published.)

IRBs and other similar ethical review bodies comprise a designated group of people trained to review and oversee a wide range of projects. Their goal is to focus on the ethics of the work and safety of study participants. Unlike many other health research studies, ethnographic studies often have more engagement in the field and with study participants, and IRB reviewers may be less familiar with the specific risks and benefits of ethnographic work. When proposing ethnographic work to the IRB, it is critical to proactively think through what the IRB will want to know and how to frame the necessary information (see Box 2.2).

IRBs may have dozens of forms, including those detailing how sites are selected, how participants are identified and recruited, the informed consent process, and how data are stored. While it is necessary to complete the required forms, the overriding goal is to be ethical. How will the research team act to responsibly and proactively protect study participants and settings?

Box 2.2 Strategies to get an ethnographic study approved by an IRB

- Find a model.
  - Ask colleagues for examples of ethnographic studies that have received IRB approval.
- Speak with an IRB representative early on.
  - Bring questions, especially about sections of the forms that may not align directly with your protocol.
  - Ask questions to ensure understanding of their key concerns and priorities.
- Use the study design details (see Table 2.5).
  - Who will be engaged in the research?
  - Whom and what will be observed/not observed, and how will observations be done?
  - What might you learn?
  - What are the potentially unsafe situations; how will you know, and when should you act and how?

Specifying the participants in ethnographic research

An issue often unique to ethnographic research is who the participants are and how they might be involved. Ethnographies might include community members as advisors instead of research participants or observation of specific people in a highly populated area (e.g., a healthcare clinic). Specify the different people who might be encountered and how the research team will interact with people (if at all). For example, if the research team is observing people in the emergency department, the protocol needs to be specific about who is being observed, who is not being observed, what data are recorded, and if any identifiable information is being collected (and if so, how this information will be protected and stored). An excerpt of an IRB protocol detailing who will be observed and what will be recorded is provided in Box 2.3, along with the data collection instrument in Box 2.4.

Box 2.3 Example of IRB study protocol describing observation

Purpose: To characterize how patients, staff, and clinicians currently interact with the My HealtheVet (MHV) Clinical Reminder, with the goal of developing a program to enhance the ability of the staff and clinicians to support patients' enrollment and authentication in MHV.

Protocol

- Prior to day of planned observation: observer meets with clinic supervisor/leadership to explain the observation process and arranges day(s) and time(s) to visit.
- Day of visit: observer explains the process to the staff member(s) and clinician(s) to be observed and obtains voluntary consent.
- Who is being observed:
  - Only the employee who gave consent will be followed.
  - Patients are observed during the typical interaction during which the MHV clinical reminder is addressed; this interaction may include discussion regarding other clinical reminders and the assessment of vital signs. Verbal consent from patients is obtained by the care provider.
- Observation notes will be recorded on a worksheet.
  - Observation worksheets will be stored in a locked cabinet.
  - No personal health information (PHI) will be collected.
- At any time, the patient or staff member, or anyone who interacts with them, may ask the observer to leave the area and/or stop recording notes. The observer will respond to this request immediately.
- Where observations will take place:
  - Participants will be observed as they perform their usual, work-related activities.
  - Participants will not be followed into private areas such as the restroom or dressing room.
  - Multiple clinical reminders are typically addressed in the same clinical encounter, along with the collection of patient vital signs. To limit disruption to the patient visit, the observer will remain during the entire pre-provider appointment with the health tech or nurse, unless requested to leave by either the patient or caregiver.

- We will not record information that is not relevant to the development of an intervention to enhance MHV registration.
  - The MHV Clinical Reminder induces two questions and some education/motivation about MHV. We will record answers to the questions and key phrases from the related conversation about MHV, as well as any nonverbal communication that may occur.
  - Specific responses to other clinical reminders, vitals results, and discussion unrelated to MHV are irrelevant to the study and will not be recorded in any way. However, the *process* by which the staff and veteran interact in satisfying these reminders may be relevant, especially if the process differs from reminder to reminder. Therefore, we will ascertain information about the process, the communication, the timing, and their relationship to the workflow of the visit.

Box 2.4 Example description of observation data collection provided to IRB

The following is a general outline of the information we intend to collect. Observers will remain alert to any interactions or behaviors in the primary care setting that may be relevant to developing an intervention in primary care to support the enrollment of patients in My HealtheVet (MHV):

(1) Time to do all clinical reminders asked (minutes)
(2) Time spent on MHV reminder specifically
(3) Results—how many patients had internet? How many were already signed up for MHV?
(4) If have internet and not registered already: key phrases used during education of MHV
(5) Patient responses
    (a) Questions and reaction to the education of MHV
    (b) Indication of commitment or disinterest
(6) Caregiver education and responses
    (a) Key phrases used to educate or motivate
    (b) Materials given and/or actions taken
(7) Problems and/or interruptions
(8) General comments from staff

Ethnographic research sometimes involves key end-users or community members as advisors instead of research participants. How these end users or community members will be involved in data collection and/or analysis should also be specified. For example, will the community member be involved in recruitment, informed consent, and/or data collection? Will the community member have access to identifiable data? Think through the roles these individuals will have on the team, the training they will require, and how they are expected to contribute. This specification will be essential for the research team, the community members, and the IRB.

IRBs typically require a research protocol detailing each step of the research plan, including: how participants are identified, recruited, and consented; how data will be collected; how data are stored; and with whom it can be shared. Writing the research protocol is an opportunity to think through the range of scenarios for each of these steps.

Box 2.5 Example: Minimizing risks to participants and team members

- *Participants' safety*
  - All research team members will receive training on identifying issues and how to respond to and report incidents.
  - If we learn of things that might be dangerous to patients or others, such as imminent danger or intent to harm, the research team will report this to the site's HIV Clinic point of contact.
  - If at any time during a telephone or in-person interview the patient becomes distressed, we will refer them to the patient crisis line (1-800-xxx-xxxx).
- *Research Team members' safety.* During the in-person, off-site interview, additional safety procedures will be put in place to protect the research team.
  - When scheduling the interview, we will review the interview process, including a safety checklist.
  - The safety checklist will include items such as who else might be in the home, whether there will be pets present, how to access the home, and where to park.
  - Two research team members will go to each in-person interview.
  - The team will try to schedule the interview during the day.
  - The location of the interview will be left with other members of the research team.
  - The team will bring their cell phones.
  - At the beginning and end of the interview, the research team will notify another team member letting them know the interview has started/ended.
  - If the research team observes things that raise concerns about their safety, they will immediately end the interview and leave.
  - Safety phrase. If a member of the research team is concerned about safety during an in-person interview, one of us will call another team member and say, "I left the blue folder." This will let the team know we believe we are in danger, and they should call the police.
  - The research team dress code includes avoiding expensive or extravagant items, wearing comfortable shoes, not valuables, and limiting the amount of cash carried.
  - No research team member will enter a home if they feel unsafe.

Risks to participants or research team

Ethnographic research takes place in real-world settings. The focus of health-related ethnographies might be people with serious illnesses, difficult life experiences, or even seemingly mundane or routine provision of healthcare services that could become unexpectedly tense. Any of these individuals or settings could raise issues that require attention, such as an unmet healthcare need or imminent concern (e.g., suicidal ideation or intent). Further, the real-world setting can create unique challenges for study team members. Before starting data collection, a research team should think through possible challenges and ways to keep both participants and research team members safe (Box 2.5).

Dealing with setbacks

Ethnography happens in real-world settings. Issues should be expected, and even anticipated. Problems can run the gamut from political or climate events, to an obstinate person or lack of funding. Good ethnography builds in flexibility and creativity to get around these inevitable issues.

Conclusion

Designing an ethnographic study can be a creative and challenging exercise. At its core, the design is driven by the research question and the myriad perspectives that can provide insights. Specific methods can be brought together to yield a holistic, nuanced, and frequently novel view onto a perplexing healthcare problem. The early phases of designing an ethnographic study provide an opportunity to think through a range of methods, including interviews and observation, as described in further detail in Chapter 3.

Case 2

Designing an ethnographic evaluation for a substance use disorder intervention
Megan McCullough

This case study comes from an intervention evaluation that Megan and her team conducted entitled, "Leveraging Clinical Pharmacy Practitioners for Rural Veteran Access: Substance Use Disorder (CRVA-SUD)." Medications for opioid use disorder and medication-assisted treatment for alcohol use disorder are gold-standard treatments for substance use disorders (Gordon et al. 2020), yet there is a persistent national shortage of qualified providers to deliver these treatments, which can limit patient access to them, particularly in rural areas (Butryn et al. 2017; Valenstein-Mah et al. 2018). The stakes are high: in a recent study, veterans who did not receive medications for opioid use disorder had a more than fourfold increase in suicide/overdose death compared to those who did (Vakkalanka et al. 2021). Rural veterans are at a deeper disadvantage: in 2018, only 27% of rural-dwelling veterans received medications for opioid use disorder compared with 34% of urban-dwelling veterans (Gordon et al. 2020). Table 2.10 provides an overview of an ethnographic study examining substance use disorder care, including the research question, the methods, and other ethnographic features.

To address the need for access to substance use disorder care and high-quality medication-assisted treatment, the CRVA-SUD intervention hired 35 CPPs and embedded them into clinical teams to serve in mental health, pain, or primary care clinics for a three-year initiative. The CPPs were trained in the most updated approaches to substance use disorder care—including medication-assisted treatment, harm reduction, and evidence-based comprehensive medication management—in virtual bootcamps with periodic follow-up meetings and educational presentations. The CPPs were given performance metrics (e.g., number of patient encounters), support from a site champion (usually an Associate Chief of Pharmacy), mentoring (in groups or individual), and opportunities for networking with other CPPs in the program and consultative site visits if performance metrics were not being met or there were other implementation issues. Megan's team was asked to evaluate the initiative, focusing on how CPPs delivered substance use disorder care, how CPPs were integrated into their interprofessional clinical teams, how much clinicians and other team members felt that CPPs were relieving/assisting with substance use disorder patients, and CPPs' perceptions of burnout and performance metrics.

Table 2.10 Ethnographic features

Research question	*Methods*	*Other ethnographic features*
How is substance use disorder care organized and functioning across the multiple levels of medical care, from patient to clinical care team (including clinical pharmacy practitioners [CPP]) and clinician?	■ Survey of patients, clinical team members, and CPPs, with two open-ended questions per survey ■ Observation via recordings of bootcamps ■ Ethnographic fieldnotes ■ Semi-structured interviews with CPPs, patients, and other clinical team members ■ Archival data: intervention documents, steering committee meeting notes, recordings, and notes from consultative visits	■ Holistic ■ Emic perspective of patients with substance use disorder and their providers

Megan and her team started with the standard evaluation remit as stated earlier, but as anthropologists, Megan and her colleague, Tony Pomales, also sought to craft the evaluation to embrace a holistic approach. The team wanted to understand how substance use disorder care was organized and functioning across multiple levels of medical care, from patient to clinical care team (including CPP) and clinician. The evaluation team also wanted to understand the organizational culture around medication-assisted treatment and substance use disorder care and what actually happened in an appointment from CPP and interprofessional team perspectives. Furthermore, to be holistic, the team reasoned that the evaluation needed to include the "end user"—the veteran patient. What were veteran/patient perspectives on this intervention? What was it like to receive substance use disorder care from a new kind of provider? How comfortable did veterans feel with pharmacists? How effective did they feel their substance use disorder care was?

Therefore, the team chose ethnography as both a holistic study approach and a set of methods addressing comprehensive questions from multiple perspectives. In this case, the team needed to balance the needs of funders (i.e., a program office within VA tasked with supporting healthcare access for rural veterans) with conducting an evaluation using multiple qualitative methods to meet the end goal. For example, the funders were more accustomed to using quantitative approaches in evaluation and had a limited understanding of qualitative methods, so the evaluation team incorporated a survey across all participants. However, the evaluation team was also driven by other questions. We saw an opportunity to illuminate the complex interrelationships of care (including potentially insufficient care) among patients, members of the substance use disorder clinical teams/interprofessional care teams, and clinicians. This approach included the sociomedical interactions among participants, the medical hierarchy of who can assert authoritative knowledge, interprofessional clinical dynamics, and the patient/CPP relationship, as well as patient voices regarding their substance use disorder treatment desires, needs, and results. Veteran and CPP perspectives (individually and collectively) needed to be heard.

The evaluation team was able to make the case for incorporating patients' perspectives in evaluating all aspects of the treatment program directed at them. The goal was to loosen the directionality of "at patients" to capture the dynamic relationship that exists *between* CPP and patient. The evaluation team saw the treatment program as interactive and not directed from one party (CPP) to another (veteran). As a result, they explicitly sought to capture data on the kinds of dynamics and the quality of relationships veterans experienced with their CPPs in the medication-assisted treatment appointment and through substance use disorder treatment.

The team also sought to account for the complexity of change through time and the challenging nature of substance use disorder treatment. Substance use disorder treatment may be complicated by issues of stigma and the challenges of updating practice approaches within rural teams, prescribing for medication-assisted treatment, and integrating and clarifying roles among CPPs and rural teams. The team outlined an ethnographic approach involving semi-structured interviews inviting diverse perspectives—from CPPs, patients, and many different clinical team members. They developed draft interview guides, and every interview guide was reviewed by CPPs, members of their clinical teams, and patients with substance use disorder experience. Each suggestion for changes was carefully considered and many changes were made by Megan and her team. The evaluation team also designed and distributed separate surveys for patients, clinical team members, and CPPs, with two open-ended questions per survey. They also used archival data (ethnographic fieldnotes, intervention documents, steering committee meeting notes), recordings of bootcamp trainings, and notes from consultative visits. In previous studies, they had used direct observation to develop a better understanding of how CPPs work and were able to use this knowledge to inform interview guides and surveys. As the COVID pandemic overtook this project, Megan and her team were unable to pursue direct observation in person; however, they were able to observe bootcamp trainings for CPPs that were occurring virtually. The goal was to ethnographically "layer" these multiple in-depth experiences regarding medication-assisted treatment and substance use disorder care for rural veterans at every site involved in this project.

Using this holistic approach, the evaluation team learned about the complex landscape of substance use disorder treatment for rural veterans from many perspectives, which has served them well in other evaluations on CPP integration into clinical teams (McCullough et al. 2021; Zogas et al. 2021; 2023). From surveys and semi-structured interviews with clinical team members in mental health, pain, and primary care settings, the team learned that more recent best practices for substance use disorder were less frequently used in rural areas. Social workers and some rural clinicians reported that there were stigmatizing attitudes toward medication-assisted treatment itself. CPPs reported that harm reduction approaches and medication-assisted treatment were viewed as a "shortcut" or somehow less legitimate ways of treatment. Many rural healthcare clinicians and providers used stigmatizing language about veterans seeking substance use disorder treatment; for example, remarking on "dirty urine" and the desire to "fire" substance use disorder patients and remove them from programs and treatment. Some providers voiced beliefs that if a patient tested positive for marijuana they should be expelled from treatment (which was no longer VA policy) and that many opioid use disorder patients were medication-seeking and not "real" pain patients.

Some clinicians—for example, psychiatrists—appreciated CPPs' work on medication-assisted treatment. The team also heard from CPPs and other clinical team members that CRVA-SUD CPPs were essential in educating rural team members about evidence-based treatment for substance use disorder and how to deliver care in a patient-centered, non-stigmatizing manner. At the same time, CPPs reported challenges in becoming integrated into clinical teams and felt they were not always fully accepted (McCullough et al. 2021). They described educating their peers on recent approaches to substance use disorder care, feeling that veterans/patients lacked other providers who understood their struggles with substance use disorder, and a sense that few providers took the time to explain medication-assisted treatment to patients.

The team learned through interviews, archival notes, fieldnotes, and recordings of meetings that CPPs dedicated a significant amount of time to tasks such as linking their substance use disorder patients to numerous services (care coordination), messaging their patients' other providers, and identifying medication interactions. Through layering interviews, they learned that CPPs were "boundary spanners" for their patients, and they serve as clinical team members who optimize care coordination by linking internal and external networks and processes of care within their organizations. In this case, CPPs were linking their patients to appointments, to other providers for appropriate care, and to more information regarding their medications not only for opioid and alcohol use disorder treatment but also for other conditions and concerns.

More significantly, the team learned that patients deeply valued their relationship with their CPPs (McCullough et al. 2016). They saw this dyadic relationship as unique and especially caring. To illustrate these relationships, the team developed ethnographic case portraits, as seen in Figures 2.1–2.3.

Compassionate Relationship-Centered Care

Being recognized – Alex's Story

Alex – 45-year-old Veteran; triple diagnosis – PTSD, chronic pain and AUD

- Reported previous negative experience of healthcare in the community:
  - Was seeing a community provider for pain management for two years who made him feel "very insecure" and "belittled" – "He didn't recognize me."
- How CPP experience was different
  - CPP "made [him] feel comfortable discussing [his] personal, health-related matters"
  - Felt like his CPP was "genuinely concerned with [his] recovery and well-being"
  - Alex's community provider never took the time to learn his name, whereas his CPP had learned his name by their second session – "she knows me by name, greets me"
  - **What being recognized by his CPP meant to Alex: "It actually feels like they're there for me. I'm a person. I feel more comfortable feeling like a person…I feel more comfortable to open up about topics that, you know, are hard to share."**

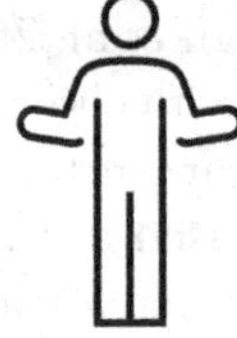

Figure 2.1 Compassionate relationship-centered care: Being recognized—Alex's story

Compassionate Relationship-Centered Care

Knowing the little things – Sandra's Story

Sandra – 33-year-old Veteran

- What she had gleaned from her years-long struggle with alcoholism:
  - Sandra: "It's hard to listen to addicts and stuff, 'cause I don't know, sometimes you hear it so much it's like, 'Yeah, yeah,' you know?"
- How CPP experience was different
  - What "helped a lot" before and after inpatient treatment was not only having someone who was effective at CMM but also "so personable"
  - Sandra: "[My CPP] actually seemed to care, you know... And it was really nice to have someone that actually listened to you and stuff and understand somebody."
  - Over a two-year period, she was able to develop a "connection" with her CPP that was helped by the way **"he would remember, you know, like how my schooling's going...like, he really remembered, like, the little stuff, you know, how my grandma was doing...So, he just made it very, very personable."**

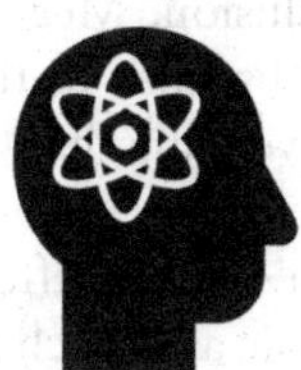

Figure 2.2 Compassionate relationship-centered care: Knowing the little things—Sandra's story

The evaluation team's ethnographic approach revealed nuanced data from many perspectives. In health services and social science literature, the "healing dynamic" is often imagined as a clinician-patient dyad. But in this era of interprofessional team care and a contraction of available primary care and internal medicine clinicians, patients have clinical/healthcare relationships with many other kinds of clinicians and providers. And, as Arthur Kleinman noted (1988), the clinical experience for patients stretches from parking lot to check-in to the taking of vitals to clinician interactions. The veteran interview data showed that their interactions with CPPs were critical. Veterans noted that CPPs "care about caring" and that manifests in the ways that CPPs use relational practices and knowledge to establish genuine connections with their patients and produce

Compassionate Relationship-Centered Care

Making time – Scott's Story

Scott – 40-year-old Army Veteran

- Reported using alcohol to "mask [his] emotional and physical pain"
- Reported previous negative experience of healthcare at VA:
  - "[My PTSD counselor] would get phone calls and would answer phone calls multiple times during our sessions together and be on the phone for extended periods of time....I didn't believe that I was being taken seriously because you're not devoting your undivided attention to me, so I'm not even gonna waste time being here."
- How CPP experience was different
  - Reported feeling a "sense of relief" because of "the service that [his CPP] provided, like, you know, she's caring."
  - **Was able to be "very open" and "honest" because his CPP was present during their sessions and made time for him "to explain and talk about the things that [he] was going through...I could let down my guard and allow myself to be vulnerable."**

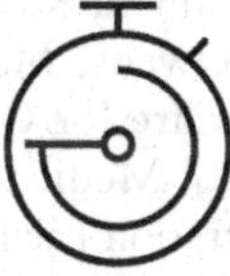

Figure 2.3 Compassionate relationship-centered care: Making time—Scott's story

trust and acceptance. Veterans emphasized that too often they, as individuals struggling with addiction and mental health issues, are treated with less respect and stigmatized by healthcare providers. CPPs can play a key role in repairing the harm inflicted by stigma in the past for veterans. Many rural clinicians reported that CPPs, with their more up-to-date knowledge of substance use disorder treatment and harm reduction approaches, became educators and leaders in the treatment of substance use disorder at their sites.

In conclusion, Megan and her team found that an ethnographic approach added depth and breadth to their evaluation. Acknowledging that CPPs, clinical team members, and veterans had very different perspectives allowed them to more fully reveal the intervention's impacts, both in terms of the unexpected activities that CPPs were engaged in and the effectiveness of their patient care. Megan's team found that their ethnographic approach helped them to have insight into multiple viewpoints and multi-leveled sociocultural organizational aspects of how sites adopted CPPs as a venue for delivering full medication-assisted treatment to veterans. Their funders and operational partners embraced their ethnographic approach and incorporated results into their next substance use disorder/medication-assisted treatment intervention, integrating mental health into substance use disorder care.

References

Butryn, Tracy, Leah Bryant, Christine Marchionni, and Farhad Sholevar. 2017. "The Shortage of Psychiatrists and Other Mental Health Providers: Causes, Current State, and Potential Solutions." *International Journal of Academic Medicine* 3 (1): 5. https://doi.org/10.4103/IJAM.IJAM_49_17.

Damschroder, Laura J., Caitlin M. Reardon, Marilla A. Opra Widerquist, and Julie Lowery. 2022. "The Updated Consolidated Framework for Implementation Research Based on User Feedback." *Implementation Science* 17 (1): 75. https://doi.org/10.1186/s13012-022-01245-0.

Fix, Gemmae M. 2008. *When the Patient Goes Home: Understanding Recovery from Heart Surgery*. Buffalo, NY: State University of New York at Buffalo.

Fix, Gemmae M., and Barbara G. Bokhour. 2012. "Understanding the Context of Patient Experiences in Order to Explore Adherence to Secondary Prevention Guidelines after Heart Surgery." *Chronic Illness* 8 (4): 265–77. https://doi.org/10.1177/1742395312441037.

Gertner, Alex K., Joshua Franklin, Isabel Roth, Gracelyn H. Cruden, Amber D. Haley, Erin P. Finley, Alison B. Hamilton, Lawrence A. Palinkas, and Byron J. Powell. 2021. "A Scoping Review of the Use of Ethnographic Approaches in Implementation Research and Recommendations for Reporting." *Implementation Research and Practice* 2 (January): 263348952199274. https://doi.org/10.1177/2633489521992743.

Glaser, Barney G., and Anselm Strauss. 1967. *The Discovery of Grounded Theory: Strategies for Qualitative Research*. New York: Aldine Transaction.

Gordon, Adam J., Karen Drexler, Eric J. Hawkins, Jennifer Burden, Nodira K. Codell, Amy Mhatre-Owens, Matthew T. Dungan, and Hildi Hagedorn. 2020. "Article Commentary: Stepped Care for Opioid Use Disorder Train the Trainer (SCOUTT) Initiative: Expanding Access to Medication Treatment for Opioid Use Disorder within Veterans Health Administration Facilities." *Substance Abuse* 41 (3): 275–82. https://doi.org/10.1080/08897077.2020.1787299.

Hamilton, Alison B., Erin P. Finley, Bevanne Bean-Mayberry, Ariel Lang, Sally G. Haskell, Tannaz Moin, Melissa M. Farmer, and the EMPOWER QUERI Team. 2023. "Enhancing Mental and Physical Health of Women through Engagement and Retention (EMPOWER) 2.0 QUERI: Study Protocol for a Cluster-Randomized Hybrid Type 3 Effectiveness-Implementation Trial." *Implementation Science Communications* 4 (1): 23. https://doi.org/10.1186/s43058-022-00389-w.

Hennink, Monique, and Bonnie N. Kaiser. 2022. "Sample Sizes for Saturation in Qualitative Research: A Systematic Review of Empirical Tests." *Social Science & Medicine (1982)* 292 (January): 114523. https://doi.org/10.1016/j.socscimed.2021.114523.

Huynh, Alexis K., Alison B. Hamilton, Melissa M. Farmer, Bevanne Bean-Mayberry, Shannon Wiltsey Stirman, Tannaz Moin, and Erin P. Finley. 2018. "A Pragmatic Approach to Guide Implementation Evaluation Research: Strategy Mapping for Complex Interventions." *Frontiers in Public Health* 6 (May): 134. https://doi.org/10.3389/fpubh.2018.00134.

Kleinman, Arthur. 1988. *The Illness Narratives*. New York: Basic Books.

Malterud, Kirsti, Volkert Dirk Siersma, and Ann Dorrit Guassora. 2016. "Sample Size in Qualitative Interview Studies: Guided by Information Power." *Qualitative Health Research* 26 (13): 1753–60. https://doi.org/10.1177/1049732315617444.

McCullough, Megan B., Beth Ann Petrakis, Christopher Gillespie, Jeffrey L. Solomon, Angela M. Park, Heather Ourth, Anthony Morreale, and Adam J. Rose. 2016. "Knowing the Patient: A Qualitative Study on Care-Taking and the Clinical Pharmacist-Patient Relationship." *Research in Social and Administrative Pharmacy* 12 (1): 78–90. https://doi.org/10.1016/j.sapharm.2015.04.005.

McCullough, Megan B., Anna Zogas, Chris Gillespie, Felicia Kleinberg, Joel I. Reisman, Ndindam Ndiwane, Michael H. Tran, Heather L. Ourth, Anthony P. Morreale, and Donald R. Miller. 2021. "Introducing Clinical Pharmacy Specialists into Interprofessional Primary Care Teams: Assessing Pharmacists' Team Integration and Access to Care for Rural Patients." *Medicine* 100 (38): e26689. https://doi.org/10.1097/MD.0000000000026689.

McElroy, Ann, and Patricia K. Townsend. 2014. *Medical Anthropology in Ecological Perspective*, 6th ed. Boulder, CO: Westview Press, a member of the Perseus Books Group.

Morse, Janice M., Michael Barrett, Maria Mayan, Karin Olson, and Jude Spiers. 2002. "Verification Strategies for Establishing Reliability and Validity in Qualitative Research." *International Journal of Qualitative Methods* 1(2): 13–22.

Nelson, James. 2017. "Using Conceptual Depth Criteria: Addressing the Challenge of Reaching Saturation in Qualitative Research." *Qualitative Research* 17 (5): 554–70. https://doi.org/10.1177/1468794116679873.

Vakkalanka, Priyanka, Brian C. Lund, Stephan Arndt, William Field, Mary Charlton, Marcia M. Ward, and Ryan M. Carnahan. 2021. "Association between Buprenorphine for Opioid Use Disorder and Mortality Risk." *American Journal of Preventive Medicine* 61 (3): 418–27. https://doi.org/10.1016/j.amepre.2021.02.026.

Valenstein-Mah, Helen, Hildi Hagedorn, Chad L. Kay, Melissa L. Christopher, and Adam J. Gordon. 2018. "Underutilization of the Current Clinical Capacity to Provide Buprenorphine Treatment for Opioid Use Disorders within the Veterans Health Administration." *Substance Abuse* 39 (3): 286–88. https://doi.org/10.1080/08897077.2018.1509251.

Vasileiou, Konstantina, Julie Barnett, Susan Thorpe, and Terry Young. 2018. "Characterising and Justifying Sample Size Sufficiency in Interview-Based Studies: Systematic Analysis of Qualitative Health Research over a 15-Year Period." *BMC Medical Research Methodology* 18 (1): 148. https://doi.org/10.1186/s12874-018-0594-7.

Zogas, Anna, Chris Gillespie, Felicia Kleinberg, Joel I. Reisman, Ndindam Ndiwane, Michael H. Tran, Heather L. Ourth, Anthony P. Morreale, Donald R. Miller, and Megan B. McCullough. 2021. "Clinical Pharmacist Integration into Veterans' Primary Care: Team Members Perspectives." *The Journal of the American Board of Family Medicine* 34 (2): 320–27. https://doi.org/10.3122/jabfm.2021.02.200328.

Zogas, Anna, Chris Gillespie, Felicia Kleinberg, Joel Reisman, Ndindam Ndiwane, Michael Tran, Heather Ourth, Anthony Morreale, Donald Miller, and Megan McCullough. 2023. "Clinical Pharmacy Practitioners' Semi-Visible Labor: Building Referral Relationships in Interprofessional Collaborative Care." *Journal of Interprofessional Care* 37 (5): 698–705. https://doi.org/10.1080/13561820.2023.2169665.

CHAPTER 3

Conducting pragmatic ethnography in healthcare research

Introduction

Using ethnography as a methodological approach can pose unique challenges, particularly in healthcare research, so this chapter offers practical guidance for real-world data collection. First, we discuss where ethnography happens and how to build the kinds of clinic- and community-based partnerships that make ethnography possible. Because observation can be a defining strength of ethnographic approaches, we provide suggestions for doing observation and using fieldnotes and other strategies to document what is seen and learned. Because so much of healthcare research occurs in interdisciplinary teams, we also discuss best practices for team-based ethnography, including strategies for ensuring a consistent-but-flexible approach among team members and bringing together insights that reflect diverse vantage points. We offer lessons learned in retaining rigor throughout the data collection process and keeping plans for analysis front of mind in order to ensure data collection remains focused and on-target.

Where ethnography happens

As anthropologists and social scientists have shown over the past century, ethnography can occur in any environment where people live, work, play, or gather. Environments where healthcare or other social services are provided can be particularly salient for ethnographic work because they generally feature complex cooperation and communication among a variety of people, organized around a shared intention to increase health and reduce suffering (Pope 2005). The stakes of social organization and sensemaking in these settings are often high.

In 2007, Erin began conducting an ethnographic study in San Antonio, Texas, focused on understanding experiences of posttraumatic stress disorder (PTSD) among US veterans of the then-raging conflicts in Iraq and Afghanistan. One of the settings for this ethnography was a VA specialty care clinic focused on delivering PTSD care to veterans of all eras, from World War II, Korea, and Vietnam, as well as to the newer

DOI: 10.4324/9781003390657-3

generation returning home. For many years, the clinic's psychiatrists, psychologists, and social workers had offered an array of individual and group therapy options, largely based in psychodynamic principles of therapeutic rapport, open communication, and talking through thoughts and feelings. Support groups had, in many cases, been serving the same veterans for a decade (or more), and providers often spoke of the relationships they had built with individual veterans, and the gains they had seen those veterans experience over time. Yet during the time that Erin was based in the clinic, a new set of evidence-based psychotherapies was introduced, emphasizing time-limited (typically 12-week) therapies built around principles of cognitive behavioral therapy and the need for directly remembering and talking or writing about traumatic memories. Rather than initiating a simple shift in treatment practices, the new therapies prompted a lengthy period of soul-searching and some conflict among clinic providers, who saw the new therapies in diverse ways. Some viewed the new treatments as bordering on unethical, because of their brief duration and direct confrontation with trauma. Others viewed them as promising and potentially revolutionary, believing they offered a more effective set of tools for improving the quality of veterans' lives.

From a methodological standpoint, Erin was struck by how different methods in her ethnography revealed different facets of the conflict. In individual interviews, clinicians revealed their own perspectives on the shifting treatment norms, usually framed within their past histories of training and experience. In observation of staff meetings, she saw that providers expressed similar perspectives, but emotions ran higher and debate was frequent. The most potent language was typically seen in casual conversations occurring in the clinic's less formal spaces, like the coffee lounge. Integration of these methods as ethnography revealed a shifting and multifaceted portrait of the changes occurring in how providers viewed and sought to heal the aftermath of trauma.

In another example, led by Carolyn Tarrant and other researchers (2016) in the United Kingdom, the study team was interested in better understanding how hospitals in Scotland were implementing a treatment bundle for sepsis. The treatment bundle called for six steps to occur within the first hour after identifying a case of sepsis (e.g., administering oxygen, taking blood cultures). The ethnographic team conducted some 300 hours of nonparticipant observation, documented through fieldnotes, and accompanied by semi-structured interviews of providers, and found that the six steps were not happening as intended. The problem was not one of provider attitudes or behavior—the inpatient nurses and physicians agreed that the bundle was valuable and effective and they were trying to go through the six steps. Where they ran into trouble was how frequently each of the six steps required coordinating with other members of the team—on a busy ward, with other patients needing care, and with team members moving separately around throughout the area. In this case, ethnography laid bare the real-world challenges of implementing the treatment bundle and suggested new strategies for improving how sepsis care was delivered.

In both of these examples, ethnographic work was occurring in clinical spaces, but nearly any space can be ethnographic: a street corner, a park, an auditorium, a field, or a home. Healthcare settings may feature both public and private spaces, such as the centralized desks of providers, nurses, and clerks, which frequently function as gathering hubs where people enter and exit between activities, as well as the private spaces of clinic rooms and offices (Greenhalgh and Swinglehurst 2011). Home- and community-based settings may likewise vary in being public or private, offering unique opportunities for understanding the worlds and experiences of participants (Pilbeam, Greenhalgh, and Potter 2023). Different methods are better suited to different spaces. For example, individual interviews typically work best in spaces where there is privacy and the conversation can be uninterrupted, allowing the participant to feel at ease sharing their views and experiences and creating the opportunity for a more free-flowing discussion. By contrast, observational methods inherently require there be some activity or interaction to observe, although this can vary from observing how an individual interacts with technology to observing a one-on-one clinical interaction to observing how clinical team members converse, coordinate, and move around in a busy hospital ward. When thinking about data collection in healthcare research, it can be valuable to think about where critical conversations, events, and decisions are occurring, which are directly observable, and how data collection will be organized to bring together multiple perspectives on *what is happening and why* in the physical and social settings most relevant to the research question.

Building ethnographic partnerships: Trust, reflexivity, and power

Conducting ethnography often requires gaining entry into new settings and environments, and typically that necessitates reaching out to build relationships with the clinic-and/or community-based partners who can make that possible, whether by making introductions to key points of contact, serving as a liaison to a new group of participants, or formally granting permission. As ethnography and other community-engaged and participatory approaches have increasingly gained traction in healthcare, social science, and even consumer research, growing attention has been paid to the importance of these partnerships and strategies for building and maintaining them (Finley et al. 2024). Outreach to invite a new partnership may be as simple as a phone call or email of introduction, but establishing credibility and trust with new partners takes time and can benefit from being mindful of a few core principles. At the most basic level, it is essential to be authentic, respectful, and transparent. If the researcher is interested in conducting an ethnographic study to better understand how shared decision-making is negotiated in an orthopedic surgery clinic, then that goal should be made clear in early outreach efforts. The researcher should be direct in communicating what participation in the project might look like, what input and activities will be requested from participants, and how study findings will be used and communicated, including back to the partners themselves. If the research is taking a more participatory approach, as in the case studies that follow this chapter, with the expectation that study methods and focus will evolve to reflect partner perspectives and feedback, that should also be stated directly.

After the initial outreach, it may take significant time to establish credibility and, later, meaningful trust with new partners. Suggested strategies for building trust in new partnerships include engaging in frequent interactions; demonstrating empathy, expertise, and responsiveness to a partner's priorities and concerns; and a commitment to bi-directional communication and co-learning (Himmelman 2002; Metz et al. 2022). There is no substitute for continuing to show up and demonstrate commitment to shared goals over time.

Ethnography, as with all qualitative research, also requires researchers to engage in thoughtful reflexivity, critically examining how their social and embodied selves—

including gender, class, education, ethnicity, sexual orientation, life experience, etc.—may affect their relationships with partners and participants in research and with what implications for shaping findings and study impact (Rankl, Johnson, and Vindrola-Padros 2021; Richards and Emslie 2000). For example, as a white cisgender woman who began her career studying masculinity among Anglo and Latino combat veterans in South Texas, Erin learned to be attentive to how gender and ethnicity shaped interactions with participants. Maintaining a sense of reflexivity is much like practicing mindfulness, in that thoughtful attention can allow us to see our interactions more clearly and can open up new insights and wiser responses to what is happening around us (Kornfield 2009).

Power is an important piece of both reflexivity and establishing relationships (Finley et al. 2023); often the research team has relatively high social power within a clinical or community setting, but that is not always the case. Where the researcher has relatively high power, addressing and leveling power differentials can support increased trust and psychological safety (Metz et al. 2022). This not only increases the authenticity of the research partnership but is also likely to increase the trustworthiness of the resulting data. People usually tell the clearest truths when it feels most safe to do so. Where the researcher has relatively little power, it is important to pay attention to the relevant hierarchies and work within them in a way that will allow for gaining credibility over time (Shattuck et al. 2022). Aijazi and colleagues (2021) have described how power was experienced by the different members of a team conducting collaborative research in the aftermath of an earthquake in Nepal; as told by each of the team's members, relations of power and knowledge impacted everything from how participants told their stories to whom data was gathered from. Reflexively examining our positionality as researchers is both a critical part of ethical practice and essential to achieving valid, trustworthy data.

Observation

Observation is one of the less commonly employed methods in healthcare research and yet can provide extraordinary insight. Observation can allow us to observe behaviors, locations, and systems through the lens of how people act and communicate, how roles are organized and coordinated, and who congregates where. Fix et al. (2022) point out that observational methods can be used to explore "patient or provider behaviors, interactions, teamwork, clinical processes, or spatial arrangements." Attending to appearance, verbal and nonverbal interactions, and movement patterns can reveal much about the norms and relations of a given environment.

Moreover, while methods like interviewing rely on what participants tell us, observation reveals the frequent gaps between what people say and what they do (Stuckey et al. 2014). Qualitative interviewing based on self-report is inherently limited by what our interlocutors are willing and able to articulate. Asking people to describe how or why they do things can be like asking a fish to describe swimming in water—there is so much that, as humans, we take for granted about our environments and how we move through them. A nurse entering data into an electronic medical record may be so accustomed to the process that, in describing it, he skips over critical steps he no longer notices. An individual describing their nutritional intake may forget or minimize less healthy choices. Observation can provide an opportunity to witness what is unnoticed, unreported, taken for granted, or simply uncomfortable to discuss.

Box 3.1 Participant and nonparticipant observation

- *Participant observation*: engaging as an active participant in day-to-day activities, traditionally as a resident or member of the community; may involve observing discussions and processes occurring as part of one's routine work.
- *Nonparticipant observation*: conducting naturalistic observation without actively engaging in the discussions or events under study.

There are several different types of observation commonly used in ethnographic approaches (see Box 3.1). In traditional ethnography, anthropologists rely on an ideal of participant observation, attempting to reside in and become part of a community and observing events and phenomena over time as a participant in those events. Healthcare providers and researchers embedded in healthcare systems may practice contemporary forms of participant observation today, observing discussions or processes in which they normally participate as part of their routine work (Palinkas and Zatzick 2019). However, nonparticipant observation is increasingly common, particularly in clinical settings where the researcher may not have the skills or training to participate directly. This may involve sitting in on critical meetings or discussions, or observing key behaviors and interactions, as an acknowledged but nonparticipant presence. In both cases, the first responsibility of the observer is to ensure that others present have an understanding of the research and what it entails, what is being observed, and how the information will be used; they should also have provided appropriate consent.

It is interesting that while ethnographic observation runs the risk of bias from the Hawthorne Effect, in which people shift their behavior when they are aware of being observed, ethnographic data are generally less subject to this bias precisely because they are gathered over time. As trust in the ethnographic partnership grows, those observed are more likely to relax into more authentic (less self-conscious) patterns of speech and behavior (Monahan and Fisher 2010).

An essential first step in any collaborative research is building the research team. For direct observation, the team should ideally be multidisciplinary and inclusive of community members. It should include at least two observers, at least one of whom has prior experience with observation (Fix et al. 2022). As seen in the case studies that follow this chapter, including diverse training and experiences on the team can help in establishing trust and credibility with sites and can support more nuanced interpretations of the data once gathered. Including multiple observers can help to ensure that observation is focused and comprehensive, particularly when observers remind each other to notice and document phenomena in a complete and consistent way.

In Chapter 2, we discuss selecting what will be observed as part of the ethnographic study design. Perhaps the most critical decision point is whether observation will be continuous, extending over a period of time, or focused, narrowing in on specific events. For example, studying the delivery of cancer care at an academic institution, one might plan to spend two months conducting continuous ethnography in the clinical setting, observing patient visits, cancer team consultations, etc., and exploring key processes, practices, and challenges emerging across diverse interactions. Alternatively, in a more focused ethnography, one might opt to observe a series of 20 cancer team consultations, with the goal of specifically examining how multidisciplinary teams come to consensus around treatment recommendations. Focused ethnography tends to be applied and pragmatic, targeted and problem-focused, gathering more structured data on preselected topics (Bikker et al. 2017; Higginbottom, Pillay, and Boadu 2015). In making use of more targeted and structured data collection, focused ethnography has the added benefit of increasing the comparability of data gathered across sites and by multiple observers.

Fieldnotes and other methods of documenting observation

Observation and data collection tools (e.g., fieldnotes) go hand-in-hand, as documentation allows observations to be captured and recorded for later analysis. Whether observation will be continuous or focused, it is essential to determine what will be observed, when, and how, and to develop data collection tools to support systematic documentation (see Box 3.2). For example, if a specific behavior—for example, handwashing on an inpatient unit—is the focus of observation, it may be helpful to develop a structured form for capturing how frequently handwashing occurs, under what circumstances (e.g., after leaving a patient's room), whether it was completed as recommended (e.g., using a specific soap for the recommended length of time), etc. (Goedken et al. 2019). Observation in ethnography is commonly documented via some form of fieldnotes. Fieldnotes provide a detailed written description of verbal or nonverbal events, experiences, or encounters. They may run the gamut from relatively unstructured to highly structured, depending on the research goals, familiarity with what is being observed, and the training and skills of the team.

Unstructured fieldnotes may be as simple as a detailed narrative description of the observation event and may be appropriate for an exploratory research project. In her ethnographic study of veterans with PTSD, Erin wrote many hundreds of pages of fieldnotes describing observations made in the clinic, visits to community events and people's homes, and conversations occurring outside the bounded limits of formal interviews (see Box 3.3). In contrast, unstructured notes are unlikely to be a good fit for team-based ethnography. Because what we observe is so profoundly shaped by our own expectations, histories, and biases, unstructured notes contributed by multiple team members are likely to be so idiosyncratic that they become difficult to analyze. At minimum, Fetters and

Box 3.2 Practical tips for observation

- Phenomena to be observed must occur in accessible settings and frequently enough for observation to be practical.
- Phenomena to be observed should be clearly defined (who, what, when, where, and how).
- Data collection tools (e.g., fieldnotes, semi-structured or structured templates) should be tailored to address research questions and support systematic documentation across team members and observation events.
- All data collection tools should be piloted before initiating formal data collection and should maintain clear distinction between observed events and the observer's interpretations/reflections.

Box 3.3 Sample of unstructured fieldnotes

(Excerpt with permission from Finley 2011)

When I arrived at the event [Congressional Town Hall, San Antonio], held in a large auditorium at a local university, I made my way past a handful of official-looking young staffers to find [Steve and Ellen] perched in one of the upper rows of the packed theater, crowded in among several hundred other veterans and family members. Steve was in his motorized chair that day… Ellen sat beside him on her own walker, an energy drink clutched tightly in one thin and freckled hand.

I said hello to Steve, and Ellen and I chatted as the forum began. Each of the congressmen was introduced, and then three local representatives each took the podium and gave brief comments, leading up to what was clearly intended to be a keynote presentation by Rep. Bob Filner, [then] chairman of the House Committee on Veterans' Affairs. The local representatives pointed out a series of problems with VA services … including gaps in VA health care related to the influx of [Iraq/Afghanistan] veterans and the need to develop appropriate care systems for dealing with PTSD and traumatic brain injury. Each congressman made a case for his own track record in standing up for veterans… When his turn came, Chairman Filner got up and was greeted with a standing ovation. He said his thanks and then pointed out that getting four congressmen in the same room for an event like this was a rarity, calling the occasion evidence of their 'unity on behalf of all veterans.' This prompted another round of applause….

Rubinstein (2019) recommend that even relatively unstructured observation templates prompt for descriptions of the "3 Cs": *context*, or the circumstances under which observation is occurring; *content*, what happened/was observed; and *concepts*, preliminary reflections or interpretations regarding what was observed. In the case study from Dr. Gala True that follows this chapter, Gala's team used this approach to develop a semi-structured fieldnote template to capture observations at gun shows and firearm retailer events, as part of ethnographic work to explore veteran perspectives on reducing access to lethal means in suicide prevention (see Box 3.4 and Case 3b).

Having a more structured data collection tool can make it easier to capture high-priority topics. The structure can ensure consistency in documentation across observers. This format is often well-suited to the specified research questions typically examined in healthcare research and can also be more straightforward to analyze (as we will discuss in the next chapter). In one recent study, Erin and Alison created a "call sheet" to summarize the content of regularly occurring calls happening as part of implementing a new healthcare program at multiple sites (see Box 3.5). Dedicated sections prompted research team members to take notes on who attended the call, attendees' updates on progress and new developments at each site, and discussions around problem-solving and/or planning for next steps (Hamilton et al. 2023). Clearly prompting notes on specific types of information helped a team of six different observers to capture observations with enough consistency to allow comparison across sites and over time. If the study is grounded in a particular theory or framework, or requires focused attention to specific behaviors, prompting for routine observation of those priority concepts or behaviors is likely to be valuable in maintaining consistent attention to the underlying conceptual lens.

Box 3.4 Excerpt from semi-structured fieldnote template
(VISION Study; contributed by Gala True)

Background information on observation event:

Event/Group/Community attendee(s): ______________________________

____

Location: ______________________________

Team member(s)/Meeting facilitator(s): ______________________________

____

Notetaker: ______________________ Date: ______________

Sample questions/focus topics

Framing: We want to learn from you about your views on veteran firearm suicide in our community.

- First, we want to hear more about what you know (or think) about the issue of veteran suicides in Southeast Louisiana?
- What, if anything, are you and others in your community already doing to try and prevent suicide by firearm among veterans in our communities?
- What do you think are the challenges?
- Given your concerns, what do you think are acceptable and realistic ways to reduce suicide by firearm?

Sample "Team Memo" prompts

- Who else was there?
- Thinking about why we chose this event/meeting/group, did it work out the way you thought it would, or differently?
- How did it go? How well prepared did you feel? What, if anything, could have been done differently to prepare?
- What are your "take-home" observations and thoughts?
- Who was present, and how did they know each other or interact?
- What activities (if any) were taking place?
- What did you learn that felt new?
- What did you hear or learn that you've also heard in past meetings/events?

Regardless of the format, it is important to remember that fieldnotes should make a clear distinction between the observed events and any interpretation or reflection on the part of the observer. For example, if the observed behavior was a conversation about shared decision-making between a patient and provider, the notes might read as follows: *Dr. A initiated the conversation by welcoming Mr. M into the office and saying that his test results were now available and there were a few different treatment options to consider.* It may also be appropriate to note that, for example, *Dr. A seemed a little flustered when she entered the office. The conversation with Mr. M continued for about 17 minutes, and ended somewhat abruptly when Dr. A stood up from her seat,*

Box 3.5 Excerpt from structured "call sheet" template
(EMPOWER 2.0; Hamilton et al. 2023)

Background information on observation event:

Date:____________________ Site: ____________________

Site Attendees: ______________________________________

EMPOWER Attendees: __________________________________

Site updates:

- What is happening with implementation at the moment?
- How are things going at the site (e.g., changes, challenges)?
- Other updates (e.g., any staffing changes, need to change an upcoming call, etc.)

Progress on tasks/activities since last call:

- Who has been involved? What barriers have come up?

Key questions, challenges, and potential solutions

- What are the key questions or concerns right now?
- What are some potential solutions to guide next steps?

Site next steps/planned action items ________________________________

____

____

Sample dates of key site milestones

Communication plan completed ____________________

First recruitment sample pulled ____________________

summarizing her understanding of Mr. M's treatment preferences and describing next steps (scheduling the surgery and preparatory lab tests) as she made ready to leave the room. However, because interpretations of observed events may change over time, as the ethnographer develops a deeper understanding of the problem, it is important not to embed interpretation into the write-up. For example, it would not be appropriate to say that *Dr. A rushed through the discussion and became frustrated with* Mr. M, because the observer cannot know Dr. A's internal feelings or state. It could, however, be important to make a separate note that Dr. A seemed impatient as the conversation continued, and to ask Dr. A about that later if possible. It may be that she was not frustrated with Mr. M at all, but instead was worried about another patient, bothered by something happening at home, or not feeling well.

Writing fieldnotes requires discipline and reflexivity in maintaining the clear distinction between description and interpretation. The ethnographer should describe what is observed, resisting the urge to leap prematurely to interpretation (Wolfinger 2002). The reward for maintaining this distinction is increased rigor and trustworthiness in the quality of the data, and a process that allows for understanding to evolve over time as new information emerges. Leaving separate, dedicated space on a fieldnote template for questions, reflections, or initial interpretations can be helpful. This space can invite the kind of thinking that supports early recognition of emerging patterns in the data (Fix et al. 2022).

Fieldnotes of all varieties need not be limited to text. They may also include diagrams, maps, pictures, drawings, or documents, all of which can capture critical data. For example, maps of where a specific health service is located within a community can illuminate the ease or difficulty of accessing that service for local residents. A diagram illustrating where specialized equipment (e.g., point-of-care ultrasound) is located in relation to where it needs to be used (e.g., is it stored in a separate cabinet, and if so, how far from the examination or patient rooms in which it is likely to be needed?) can inform understanding of how frequently the equipment is used in routine care encounters. Alison's team used diagrams to document where new patient-facing kiosks were located in VA mental care clinics; some clinics were able to easily locate the kiosks within existing space, some made creative use of former closets, and others had to construct new spaces to house the kiosks with adequate privacy (Cohen et al. 2013). Likewise, pictures can greatly enhance the quality of fieldnotes, capturing visual information better than narrative alone.

Before beginning observation, it is useful to pilot the observation and documentation plan. This preliminary work can help a team see if they are observing or documenting behaviors as expected and where challenges may arise in gaining access, and can ensure consistency across observers (Fix et al. 2022). We'll discuss this further in the section on team-based ethnography later.

Ethnographic interviews

Interviews in their various forms are perhaps the most commonly used tool in the qualitative research toolkit. Not all interviews are ethnographic. Yet nearly all interviews have the potential to be ethnographic (see Box 3.6) if approached with a view toward understanding insider perspectives, actions, and experiences within the holistic context of the local world(s), or what McGranahan (2015) calls an "ethnographic sensibility." This may mean one-time interviews conducted with diverse individuals involved in or impacted by a healthcare concern, but more typically means interviews conducted

Box 3.6 Common features of ethnographic interviews

- Aim to understand insider perspectives, actions, and experiences within the holistic context of the local world(s)
- May occur in a single encounter; in which case, consider: (1) allowing more time to develop trust; and (2) inviting participants to reflect on their experiences and perspectives
- May occur repeatedly with an information-rich sample of participants over time
- May be more or less structured in duration and content
- May occur as part of more informal encounters and conversations, with participant knowledge and consent
- May be documented in multiple ways, for example, recording and transcription, near-verbatim notes, or templated fieldnotes

repeatedly over time with the same group of participants. Ethnographic interviews are particularly well-suited for understanding lived experience and how embedded policies or practices are viewed and experienced at the individual level. They can thus be invaluable for developing a deep and multifaceted understanding of a given health or healthcare problem, including problems that are quite complex. They can also be indispensable for capturing change over time, which is why they are commonly used in implementation research, where achieving change in behavior and/or systems is the ultimate goal (Hamilton and Finley 2019).

Perhaps the most important thing to be aware of in designing ethnographic interviews is the extent to which they occur in the context of an existing (or newly developing) relationship. One-time interviews that aim to reach an understanding of lived experience or emic perspectives may be exploratory, phenomenological, and reflective. They may be unstructured or semi-structured, but they work best when two things set the conditions for an ethnographic conversation. First, the interviewer(s) allows a bit more time in the beginning to develop preliminary trust, for all the reasons discussed earlier around perceived safety of and respect accorded to the participant and validity of the resulting data. Second, the interviewers invite the participant to speak of their own experience in a reflective way, describing not only their experience but also their understanding of that experience and how it came about.

For example, whereas a more standard qualitative interview in health services research might invite a patient to describe their past history of seeking care for a sudden tremor in their hand, an ethnographic interview is likely to invite the participant to describe what they were worried about when their hand started trembling, whom they spoke to before they called the clinic, why they went to the provider they did, how they felt about the care they received, and what they were hesitant to tell the provider (and why). One might also ask specifically about cultural influences and pressures. This can be tricky because there may be little shared agreement on what "culture" is. On the other hand, asking about culture can also be revealing. It invites the individual to speak on what features of their cultural environment feel most salient and impactful in navigating a particular concern. One-time ethnographic interviews can allow for reaching a larger sample of participants, but the research team may need to plan for longer interviews (e.g., an hour or more) to allow for reflective conversation.

By contrast, interviews that occur repeatedly with an information-rich sample of participants over time tend to involve smaller samples and can be more or less flexible in duration and content. They occur in the context of an ethnographic partnership and allow for deepening exploration and even collaborative meaning-making (DiCicco-Bloom and Crabtree 2006), for example, by returning to questions or issues raised in prior interviews, or considering how circumstances or thinking evolve over time. Gemmae and Case 5 author Justeen Hyde helped to develop a formative evaluation using ethnographic interviews to assess the acceptability and feasibility of smartphone-enabled data collection application ("app") among veterans with experience of homelessness (McInnes et al. 2022). Interviews explored how an app might be used to capture key factors influencing housing transitions, as well as factors affecting veterans' willingness to use an app, such as readability, design, and concerns about privacy. The team identified a small set of veterans with a range of experiences of homelessness and interviewed them repeatedly. The team used a structure of what they called "rapid qualitative interviews," in both long and short formats, to gather data on specific topics (e.g., physical and mental health, use of technology). Additionally, they checked in with participants by phone a few times a week to assess how they were feeling, where they had slept, and any important events or changes in the prior few days. By combining structured inquiry on key topics with regular updates on how veterans were feeling and living, the team was able to develop—within only four weeks—a deep understanding of factors relevant to the design and approach for their smartphone-enabled study plan.

As with observations, ethnographic interviews can be documented in a variety of ways, via recording and transcription, near-verbatim notes, or templated fieldnotes. One critical feature of ethnography is that it does not always occur within the bounds of a traditional interview or focus group. Participants may make the most revealing comments when the formal conversation has ended and the group is walking down the hall to the elevator, or as a side note two days later during an unexpected encounter in the break room or church or corner store. These comments can be invaluable to capture in fieldnotes, even if only in the form of quick notes or "jottings" captured in a notebook or document kept handy for that purpose (Emerson, Fretz, and Shaw 2011). One question that can arise is whether participants expect and are comfortable with these comments being treated as data and/or shared in any resulting products. If this is ever a question, it is a good idea to ask the participant directly. Whether or not they agree, they will usually appreciate that you value their privacy, and it can be a nice way to reaffirm that this is a trustworthy relationship. Asking for permission should be handled in accordance with any study approvals, but in many cases can be as simple as reaching out to say, "I have a note about this comment you made when we were talking about [X]. I think this is an important point and I'd like to include it as part of a presentation to [audience and forum]. Would that be ok for you? Do you have any concerns about that? If it is ok, would you prefer the comment be anonymous or credited to you?" (For a rich discussion of negotiating consent in ongoing ethnographic research, see Kara et al. 2023.)

Focus groups

Although focus groups are less commonly used in ethnographic research, they can be a valuable strategy for gathering information on how group members discuss and interact around a particular topic (Hamilton and Finley 2019). In a classic article, Agar and MacDonald (1995) noted that focus group data can be contextualized with a wider array of ethnographic findings and recommended ethnographic transcript analysis as a way of understanding how participants interact and build on each other's contributions as the discussion proceeds. More recently, Blackwell (2023) has argued that focus groups can offer "ethnographic closeness" if the focus group is approached as a field site and constituted as a safe space for participants to describe and reflect on their own actions and experiences.

Patient and provider interviews

One of the practical ways the need for reflexivity plays out in healthcare research is in how we approach interviews with patients and providers. In one sense, there is not much difference: our primary goals are always to engage our participants with respect and kindness and to elicit data that is meaningful and aligned with our research questions.

At the same time, we may need to think about how the roles of the individuals we interview may suggest differences in the content of interviews, language used, or approach taken. When interviewing patients about a health concern, we are often discussing an issue of great emotional significance, something that has put them or a loved one in danger, and so it may be appropriate to foreground their experiences and choices accordingly. When interviewing providers about the same topic, they are likely to approach the same problem from a vantage point that rests more in their technical expertise, their knowledge, and their professional identity. Patients and providers may (or may not) use different language to describe their experiences and priorities and may (or may not) be concerned by power differentials in the clinical or research encounter. Interview guides and approaches should consider these potential differences in priorities, experiences, and language.

Knowledge and expertise: Maintaining a beginner's mind

Another issue that can arise, particularly in interviewing providers, leadership, and other professionals within the healthcare environment, is how much technical information the interviewer needs to be familiar with prior to beginning interviews. It is essential to have a basic understanding of the topic to be able to conduct an effective interview, particularly to be able to ask useful follow-up questions in less structured, more ethnographic interviews. For example, if interviewing a provider about treatment for type 2 diabetes, the interviewer might want to have a basic grasp of the illness, how it manifests for patients, usual treatment options, and how care is organized in the setting under study. Having this information will help to ensure that the interviewer can ask thoughtful questions.

On the other hand, an interviewer with highly specialized expertise in the topic may also face the challenge of knowing too much, which can lead to making assumptions in the moment about what the provider means by a given statement, and not following up adequately on statements that could benefit from additional explanation. The goal is always to ensure the interview paints a comprehensive picture of the topics being explored *from the participant's perspective*. Regardless of how much topical expertise the interviewer has, whether a little or a lot, it can be helpful to adopt an attitude of beginner's mind, approaching the interview with openness, humility, and curiosity, and avoiding any preconceived ideas about what the respondent is likely to say or mean (Hamilton and Finley 2019; Lofland and Lofland 1995). If there is any uncertainty about what the respondent means by a particular statement, and if it feels appropriate to do so, ask!

Periodic reflections

Periodic reflections are a kind of low-burden ethnographic interview that was developed by Alison and Erin as part of a large implementation trial (Finley et al. 2018; Hamilton et al. 2017). Their research team was in the process of implementing three evidence-based practices to improve women veterans' engagement and retention in care for prediabetes, cardiovascular disease risk, depression, and anxiety, across a variety of VA sites, and needed a pragmatic way of documenting context, events, and phenomena in real-time. Periodic reflections emerged as lightly structured conversations with members of the implementation team—including project leadership and site-based staff—that are routinely scheduled to occur monthly or bimonthly over the phone or via teleconference. These guided discussions allow for gathering up-to-date information on recent activities, any changes that have been made to the intervention or implementation plan, and updates on the local or broader environment, such as staffing, workflow, or policy changes. Reflections can be recorded and saved in file or transcript form, or can be captured using near-verbatim notes.

Periodic reflections are, in other words, a structured method for conducting repeated ethnographic interviews over the course of a project. This method can also be used to check in with patients regularly about their experience of a treatment process, or with a group of community partners about the initiative they are developing. This strategy for ethnographic interviewing cannot replace on-site observation but can allow for regular check-ins with those actively engaged in ongoing events, and for continual reflection and feedback while events are relatively fresh. There is a standard guide for periodic reflections conducted with implementation teams (see Box 3.7), but this is flexible and can be adapted to meet the needs of diverse projects. Novel questions and probes can be introduced as needed. Conducting reflections over the course of the project stands in

Box 3.7 Sample periodic reflections template (Finley et al. 2018)

Goals and Focus: These reflections are intended to provide an opportunity to check in regularly about how implementation efforts are going. Our main goal is to take a few minutes to discuss, document, and reflect on key activities, events, and changes occurring over the course of implementation.

Date: ____________________

Names: ____________________

Roles: ____________________

Notetaker: ____________________

- Status update: What are the current main activities for the project? How is it going?
- Have there been any changes to the intervention or how it's being implemented in the past month?
- Have there been any outreach or engagement efforts in the past month?
- Have you seen any recent changes in the local or national environment that you think may have an impact on the study?
- Quick check: What's going well right now? What's not going so well?
- What are the next steps going forward?

Other useful areas for discussion:

- Barriers/concerns that have arisen recently? What solutions have been tried? How is that going?
- Who have been the key people involved in recent activities, efforts, and discussions? What have been their primary concerns, hopes, and/or suggestions?
- Have there been any surprises lately, or unexpected events?
- What lessons have been learned?
- Remaining thoughts, observations, or concerns?

contrast to the kind of "post" interviews that may occur months after the fact, which run the risk of introducing greater recall bias, and lack the immediacy of observations gathered (relatively) in the moment. Reflections are ethnographic in allowing close engagement over time, supporting deepening understanding, and inviting emic perspectives from participants who may have very different perspectives on a given process or event (Finley et al. 2018).

We discuss analysis of ethnographic interviews and fieldnotes in Chapter 4, but periodic reflections, like all of the methods discussed here, have the benefit of allowing for a wide variety of analytic approaches. Ethnographic data can be analyzed in an ongoing or periodic way, or retroactively. They can be supportive of formative or summative evaluation and can be analyzed using inductive, deductive (e.g., rapid), hybrid, case study, or a variety of other qualitative approaches. They are also compatible with a variety of theoretical frameworks and can be used in a qualitative study or as part of an integrated mixed-method approach (e.g., Brunner et al. 2022).

Team-based ethnography

As noted throughout, ethnographic research in modern healthcare research is often a team sport, which offers extraordinary possibilities over what can be achieved by a single ethnographer alone. In one study of the Global Polio Eradication Initiative, an international team led by anthropologist Dr. Svea Closser conducted systematic comparative ethnography across eight sites in seven nations (Closser et al. 2016). Yet many social scientists and methodologists are trained to conduct qualitative data collection as a solo rather than a group activity. There are a few useful guidelines to keep in mind when preparing and conducting data collection as a research team (see Box 3.8).

First, it is important to start by considering the training and experience of everyone on the team, and making sure that every member who will be involved with data collection and analysis has the skill set to do so. Often team members come into a project with widely varying levels of experience, and it can be useful to think about what kind of individual- or team-based training may be needed to ensure foundational skills are in place. In one project, Bunce et al. (2014) elected to begin with a two-hour in-person training that emphasized the goals of ethnographic data collection, how to ask good questions, and learning to listen. Training sessions can provide a dedicated opportunity to begin talking through the expectations and predictable challenges of the study. After the initial training, pairing less experienced team members with more experienced

Box 3.8 Practical steps for conducting team-based ethnography

- Ensure appropriate training and ongoing support for all team members
- Develop clear agreements for roles and responsibilities
- Develop and pilot materials to support ethical and rigorous data collection and storage (e.g., structured observation templates, standard operating procedures for data management)
- Conduct regular debriefing sessions
- Engage in regular cross-checking and integration of data

Table 3.1 Common roles on an ethnographic team

Role	*Tasks and Skills*
Team Lead/Principal Investigator	Provides direction and guidance; oversees the creation and refinement of data collection tools and templates; ensures all team members have adequate training and support throughout
Project Manager	Tracks and organizes data collection; may take the lead in scheduling, sending files for transcription, etc.; helps to ensure timelines and milestones are met
Analyst(s)	Often involved in both data collection and analysis, as well as developing products; must have adequate training (and ideally experience) in collecting and analyzing qualitative data
Co-Investigators	Typically less involved in ongoing data collection; often provide feedback on data collection instruments and templates and aid in troubleshooting any challenges that arise

members can help to ensure that when questions come up, they are asked early and often; investing time in training and mentoring newer qualitative researchers are essential, as they help to ensure data are gathered with consistent quality and also help to support the growing capacity of the research team over time.

Second, the team should spend time prior to data collection discussing expectations for roles and responsibilities throughout (see Table 3.1). If observational or interviewing activities need to be scheduled, who is responsible and how will the critical information be communicated to the observer/interviewer? If more than one individual will be participating in a data collection event (e.g., an interviewer and a note-taker), roles should be agreed upon ahead of time. Ensuring expectations are clear for and fully understood by every member of the team reduces the inevitable mishaps that arise in data collection. It also smooths the day-to-day conduct of the work and ensures that those involved in data collection can focus on gathering high-quality data rather than worrying about who was supposed to be recording or what meeting was missed by whom. Speaking to the practical constraints of real-world research, Bikker et al. (2017) have described how it was necessary, as a consequence of funder feedback, to condense work intended for three full-time ethnographers into activities completed by two full-time and several part-time ethnographers, with the latter all simultaneously supporting other projects. This kind of scenario is common in our experience and only underscores the importance of ensuring clarity of roles at every step.

Similarly, most team-based research projects—of any variety—require developing materials and processes to ensure data are gathered and managed in an ethical and rigorous way. If using structured observation templates, these should be developed, discussed, and piloted with the team prior to starting data collection. The rationale behind each component of data collection should be discussed so that team members know why data are being collected in a certain way. For example, the intended purpose of each question in a semi-structured interview guide needs to be clear, so that interviewers are fully equipped to assess whether the respondent has understood the question, whether the question may need to be clarified, or whether additional follow-up may be needed to get to the question's intended purpose.

When assessing theory-related constructs as part of an interview guide or observation template, it may be helpful to include bracketed headers reminding interviewers of each question/section's core purpose/concept. In other words, we might accompany a question about how a clinic team member usually arranges for patient referral with a bracket indicating this question is intended to establish baseline practices; likewise, an observation prompt for noting who attended a specific meeting may be annotated to remind observers that these data will be used to assess what organizational roles were essential to achieving a specified goal. Building prompts into the data collection process can help to ensure the consistency and rigor of data gathered by multiple team members.

Likewise, it can be helpful to establish a written standard operating procedure for how data will be gathered and managed in compliance with ethical guidelines and research approvals. Potential headers can include preparing for data collection, gathering data, storing data, tracking the data collection event, arranging for any participant compensation that may be appropriate, etc. The larger the team, the more necessary this kind of standardization is likely to become.

Once data collection has begun, regular meetings or check-ins should be held to encourage team members to talk about any questions or challenges that have come up in data collection. Problems may arise with the interview guide or observation template, for example, a question or prompt may not be clear, resulting in confusion for respondents or the research team. The earlier these problems are identified, the more quickly the issue can be clarified and addressed without creating inconsistencies in the data. Similarly, it is important to regularly check the resulting data, either by listening to recordings or reviewing notes or other documentation. Team members may see and understand instructions and events differently, and it takes time to develop a calibrated approach. As a study proceeds and understanding across the team grows, it may be necessary to update forms and processes to reflect that evolution and to collaboratively explore new questions or topics. Team members with varied life experiences may be attuned to differing viewpoints and insights emerging in the data, and these team discussions can be a place to share, coalesce, and refine these insights (Maietta et al. 2021). Similarly, working in particularly sensitive areas or topics (e.g., trauma, terminal illness, suicide prevention) may require additional support. Continuing team communication in an environment of psychological safety is essential.

As the team is gearing up to begin research, it may be helpful to read and discuss examples of team-based ethnographic work. This activity can help the team get a preliminary sense of the kinds of issues that can arise and how other teams have managed them. The two studies mentioned in this section—Bikker et al. (2017) and Bunce et al. (2014)—both provide excellent case examples for a team to consider together.

Rapid, virtual, online, and video ethnographic approaches

As the frequency and scope of ethnographic healthcare research have expanded in recent years, so too has the variety of methods available. We briefly offer a glimpse of the growing array of strategies that can be used to gather ethnographic data in the modern world and some of the pros, cons, and challenges of tackling novel methods.

In rapid ethnographic approaches, the general goal is to gather a pre-specified set of data within a time period ranging from a few days to a few months, usually for the purpose of rapidly delivering targeted information on the local context prior to intervention or implementation. In their book on conducting rapid ethnographic assessments in global public health, anthropologists Sangaramoorthy and Kroeger (2020) detail how combining traditional ethnographic methods—such as interviews and focus groups, structured observations, mapping, and even brief surveys—can produce "rich understandings of social, economic, and policy factors that contribute to the root causes of an emerging situation and provide rapid, practical feedback to policy makers and programs." In the context of global public health, Bond et al. (2019) have developed a highly structured methodology they call "broad brush surveys," which allows for conducting a series of initially open-ended but increasingly targeted discussions and observations on-site in a local community over approximately two weeks. These broad-brush surveys result in community-level profiles that summarize the local physical environment, social organization, important networks, and community narratives relevant to the health topic and have been used in the context of preparing for HIV and tuberculosis studies.

Proposed strategies for rapid ethnography in US medical care settings likewise have combined site visits, interviews, and observations, including in collaboration with site-based providers trained to conduct clinical ethnography (Palinkas and Zatzick 2019; Reisinger, Fortney, and Reger 2021). These approaches are increasingly used in preparing to implement a novel practice or intervention in a new setting and can provide critical data on local norms, resources, and constraints that may require tailoring of the implementation effort.

In general, rapid ethnographic approaches can work well to quickly and effectively gather the kind of detailed, nuanced data that anthropologists refer to as "rich" or "thick" (Geertz 1973), but necessitate a few essential ingredients. In common with the team-based ethnographic approaches discussed earlier, rapid ethnographic studies require a clear and relatively structured data collection plan, particularly when they involve collecting data across diverse sites. They also require a well-trained team with well-developed research processes. Moreover, the research team embarking on rapid ethnographic work should also have a strong grounding foundation in the language and cultural norms of the setting; rapid approaches benefit from an initial level of cultural competence and leave little time for starting from zero familiarity (Taylor et al. 2018). Finally, the research team should have strong existing networks and relationships to facilitate rapid entry into the site and connection to key participants. In other words, rapid ethnographic approaches assume a high level of skill, competence, and connection but can offer a level of insight that other rapid assessment methods would be hard-pressed to deliver.

Virtual, online, and video ethnographies, which rely—respectively—upon data collection methods based in telecommunication, online, and video-based technologies, have also come to the forefront in recent years, particularly as the COVID-19 pandemic sped the pace of adopting remote and computer-based healthcare delivery. Virtual ethnographic methods can allow for interviews and focus groups conducted via Zoom and other platforms, as well as observing healthcare encounters or meetings (Eaves et al. 2022; Boland et al. 2022). Online methods support observing and analyzing how patients or providers describe and debate their own experiences, concerns, and priorities in social media and other online fora (Gao et al. 2022; Greene et al. 2011). And video ethnography can make use of video-recorded observations, including those played back to participants to invite their reflections, as a way of capturing normative practice and eliciting perspectives on what could be done to improve care (McHugh et al. 2022; Neuwirth et al. 2012).

In short, the emergence of an ever-growing array of technologies for health-related communication and the distribution and delivery of health care offers as-yet untapped potential for spurring innovation in the use of ethnographic methods to explore complex questions.

Conclusion: Rigor, trustworthiness, and constraint

Although each of the ethnographic data collection methods described in this chapter is accompanied by unique ethical and methodological challenges, they share core principles: seek to deeply understand diverse, multilayered perspectives; be respectful, reflexive, and rigorous in data collection; and, when working in teams, maintain communication to ensure flexibility, consistency, and coordinated effort as the study proceeds.

As we close this chapter, it is worth considering once more the nature of rigor in ethnographic research. Greenhalgh and Swinglehurst (2011) have proposed evaluating the rigor of ethnography in terms of three principles: how successfully the ethnographic team achieves *authentic* immersion in the setting; how *plausible* are the explanations achieved about the relevant phenomena and the degree to which these explanations make sense to engaged participants; and the extent to which the ethnography achieves *critical* reflection on assumptions that would otherwise be taken for granted, for example, regarding how things are done, who is empowered to make final decisions, etc. In Chapter 4, we will further describe steps for maintaining rigor throughout the process of data analysis, and in Chapter 5, we will consider how to effectively report on ethnographic research in such a way as to demonstrate the trustworthiness of findings.

Case studies 3a and 3b: Participatory approaches in pragmatic healthcare ethnography

Ethnography is an approach that fits well with centering the voices of the people and communities being studied, but it doesn't happen automatically. Both historically and today, ethnographers often uphold practices and reinforce norms of how research is done that limit the space for research participants to craft their own research questions or say what is most important in their own lives. With intention, however, ethnographic methods can be a tool for precisely those ends.

Later, Drs. Anaïs Tuepker and Gala True describe some approaches and practices they have learned to make ethnographic research more participatory. If there is a general theme, it is that success in applying a participatory approach relies on building and practicing openness and trust: in the study design, in communication, in the process of defining the communities being studied, and in the researchers' willingness to go in directions that members of those communities suggest. These case studies highlight how ethnography in healthcare research can be strengthened by participatory practices, spelling out some of the methods the authors have used for building collaborative partnerships where research is conducted for and with communities.

Case study 3a
Tending to partnerships
Anaïs Tuepker

The Tending to Partnerships (TTP) study started in 2019 as a qualitative evaluation of the implementation and impacts of a single-site, hospital-based therapeutic horticulture program for veterans in Portland, Oregon. Over time, it expanded in geographic scope to encompass approximately a dozen programs in Washington and Oregon. It also expanded outside the confines of the hospital and a narrow intervention definition to community settings where a wide range of ecotherapy programs and approaches were considered. As of 2024, the study was exploring the diverse experiences of veterans with community-based ecotherapy, as well as the experiences of community organizations offering these programs and their needs and priorities for building partnerships with healthcare systems like the VA.

Although health-focused, TTP evolved out of Anaïs' reflexive observation on her own experiences as an activist around climate issues; connecting with the community and with the natural world, aside from any policy or other "external" impacts, had unexpected benefits for her mental health. As a researcher, she wanted to explore this phenomenon in other lives and contexts, especially with veterans whose complex life stories often involved physical and social displacement and disconnection. Making sense and finding patterns within veterans' experiences using standardized measures or surveys did not feel like an approach that would yield the rich narrative data needed to develop useful insights about how to spread veteran-supportive eco-therapeutic opportunities or to build healthcare-community connections. An ethnographically informed approach, where the research team could follow people in their engagement with community activities over time and gain insights from interviews, direct observations, and other materials participants chose to share, seemed more likely to yield useful insights.

An early step in the evolution of the research project involved discussing the idea, at two different time points, with a veteran engagement group, whose members confirmed that this was an idea worth exploring. They shared stimulating insights into why time in nature might be especially healing for veterans and why framing activities as "service" was different from "therapy" and might resonate with more veterans. It is important to acknowledge that the group also offered other ideas that the research team chose not to pursue. When using participatory feedback to decide on or narrow the research focus, respecting input from advisors needs to be balanced with finding an authentic fit with the interests of the research team and communicating that openly.

The earliest phase of the study involved Anaïs and her team project manager and collaborator in the project, Dylan Waller, in interviewing veterans and VA staff who ran farming and gardening programs with a therapeutic intention alongside job and skills training components. In addition to interviews, Anaïs sometimes attended the same horticulture lessons and farming workdays, digging in the soil together before COVID and then meeting over Zoom and sharing photos of separate garden beds when the group was forced to move online during the early pandemic. During these sessions, she would not take notes, focusing instead on taking part in conversations, building trust, and observing settings and interactions that she would describe afterward in notes for herself. Similarly, she had exploratory and frank conversations during this time with community organizations that wanted to partner with the VA; they frequently expressed frustration with barriers to sharing funding and human resources in VA-community partnerships and the concomitant lack of trust and respect that this conveyed to them. This was not formal data collection for the study, but by being attentive to the context in which programs were operating, Anaïs became even more interested in understanding and supporting community-based programs and partnerships.

Direct observations often provide data for formal analysis in ethnographically informed research, but as alluded to earlier, this study's data set did not include fieldnotes from direct observations. It would have been impossible for the research team of two to build in time and resources for routine presence and direct observations from a dozen different projects. Additionally, some programs operate as "veteran-only" spaces where the presence of nonveteran researchers would change the content and dynamic; it is important to respect the spaces where researchers may not be welcome or allowed. However, direct observation strongly informs the researchers' understanding of the context of programs being studied. As was outlined in the chapter, there is no substitute for "showing up," and researchers can build relationships by attending public events (especially when invited by participants) and meeting with participants less formally when there is an opportunity to see them and their programs at work. Direct observations enriched the team's ability to describe program contexts accurately and engagingly. The team developed more in-depth knowledge of programs, for example, by attending and taking notes at community events that participant groups also attended or presented at and by reading press and social media links they shared. By considering public information in this way, they learned to see the influences and context of community-based ecotherapy from a position closer to that of their participants, and from talking informally with participants, they were better able to gauge the accuracy and relevance of such "public data." Such information often found its way into the context and background sections of reports, papers, and presentations regarding the research. Anaïs built relationships and trust in a generalized way by offering time and support to initiatives in the region, such as one focused on women veteran farmers, becoming more visible and approachable to possible participants.

In addition to interviews, recently the study began employing ripple effects mapping or REM, a participatory method of appreciative inquiry to collect data and identify findings (Chazdon et al. 2017). REM is designed to bring out the impacts from a project that are most important to people involved in it and to promote group discussion about the meaning and desired direction of shared activities. Because one of the core products of REM is an actual map or figure co-created with study participants, they have a direct role in shaping the findings of the study.

One key element directing the evolution of the project has been the team's intentional following of new leads introduced by participants, who repeatedly offered variants of "there's this other group I'm involved with …" or "We've been talking with another organization about doing a similar project." In their participatory approach, Anaïs and Dylan found expanding the scope of their work as much as feasible to follow these signals from participants was important. They learned to respond to the question, "Why haven't you talked to X group?" with curiosity instead of the defensiveness that can easily arise. Ethnography is about the study of people in communities, not as isolated individuals, so they were intentional about paying attention to where participants drew the boundaries around "who" or "what" ecotherapy for veterans includes. Additionally, they tried to remember the multiple socially constructed roles participants may hold—as veterans, as patients, as community leaders, as health professionals or researchers—and to create space for them to share their reflections from all of those positions. The study participants included several veterans who also run or facilitate ecotherapy programs for other veterans. With these participants, the study team used a variant of periodic reflections as a structured way of checking in on a regular basis on how programs were or were not serving veterans, how sustainable the work felt for them, and what was helping or hindering their partnerships with healthcare systems.

Across projects and from veterans and community organization partners, Anaïs and Dylan often heard how important it is that researchers (and clinical partners) stay in touch and answer questions or inquiries promptly and clearly. They sought to prioritize timely and honest communication, asking for input and feedback and also letting people know the limits of what they could or couldn't do in response to their requests. They asked participants at the beginning about their communication preferences and wrote their institutional review board (IRB) protocol to keep as open as possible (while still respecting necessary privacy concerns) the possibility of communicating with participants via email and phone in whatever ways and however often they chose. All participants were informed in an information sheet given to them at the beginning of the study, and reminded in conversation, that they could reach out to the research team to request a conversation or interview, or to share photos or written reflections or whatever materials they chose, at any time. Anaïs and Dylan created a project website for anyone interested to be able to learn more about the research and research team and to be able to point to a public website that enhanced their credibility; the website included their pictures and brief biographies that, in addition to their research credentials, also described the ways in which they connect with land, nature, and place.

Team and individual reflexivity practices contributed to the participatory and ethnographic approach of the project. The two TTP researchers held different gender and race identities, grew up in different regions of the United States, and were approximately ten years apart in age. They recognized that they bring a lot of different life experiences to their interactions with community partners and to their analytic process. Both were nonveterans, which they viewed as a weakness for being able to understand some of the experiences participants took for granted or struggled to put into words. Both of them trained as sociologists, which made for some common ground and language but could also create blind spots. Their team-based analytic process built in formal space for discussing how their life experiences and identities shaped their encounter with the data, and they aimed to be transparent with participants about how their experiences shaped their interests and interpretations of what they were told. For example, Anaïs often shared with participants a version of the same story that opens this case study, of how this project had its genesis in her experiences of benefiting from something akin to ecotherapy.

Over time, the research team built a formal partnership with Red Feather Ranch, one of the community groups whose staff and attendees contributed data to the study, and built relationships with the study team, through repeated conversations, interviews, REM, and informal encounters in community spaces focused on avenues for healing in nature. The research team had been reflexively honest with themselves and participants about their interest in wanting to more openly explore the roles of race, gender, and indigenous heritage and healing practices for women veterans of all backgrounds healing from trauma. These were interests of this group as well, which is run by and works with women veterans to offer Earth-based healing practices (a term the organization prefers to ecotherapy, which offers a good reminder to researchers to be flexible in both terminology and thinking, to gain insight into participants' viewpoints). Members of this organization have joined the study team, with funding extended to support their time and participation. A woman veteran who is also a professional researcher, Sari Fresquez, has meanwhile joined the "internal" study team based within the VA, adding her perspective to data analysis and study communication strategies. The goal of the current phase of the research is to develop tools to help spread the program's approach to others, especially in rural areas where the program has had some early success in reaching isolated women. Through periodic reflections and continued interviews and observations, the goal is to keep adding new layers of understanding to the study of the program's impacts. In this and other projects with a community setting, the work is already contributing new critical knowledge by shifting and broadening understanding of where health "care" legitimately happens and what healing can look like even when it's not called therapy.

As a closing reflection, Anaïs and Dylan offer one question they have sometimes been asked themselves: if research participants are there to inform data collection and analysis at (almost) every step of the way, what happens to the researcher's ability to be critical or to make observations that participants might disagree with? The answers to this question are dependent on the researcher's beliefs about the nature of knowledge, the purpose of research, and the power relations between the involved parties. Participatory ethnography's emphases on trust and transparent communication steer the researcher away from being overtly critical of participants' behaviors and beliefs, but in Anaïs' experience, this can also provide a healthy push to researchers to reflect on the cultural assumptions that underlie the tendency to critique without dialogue. Good ethnography promises to deliver new insights via critical reflection. This can mean new insights that have not before been seen or acknowledged by those *outside* the community being studied—by researchers, policymakers, or healthcare professionals. One can take seriously the premise of approaches like Popular Education and participatory action research (PAR) that people are the experts in their own lives and engage them in dialogue where retaining a "beginner's mind" can stimulate new insights, both for the formal researcher and the research participants. Participants in TPP (and other studies) have commented how they have had new insights by being asked about their experience and hearing what others, including the research team, also have to say; weaving these insights together, in dialogue, can be a profoundly rewarding and enlightening experience for the researcher.

Case study 3b

Ethnography and participatory research: Bringing in community voices

Gala True

This case study draws upon PAR conducted by VA researchers in collaboration with members of firearm-owning communities in Louisiana, including veterans and their families, firearm retailers and instructors, members of gun clubs, and attendees at gun shows. The purpose of this work, titled the Veteran-Informed Safety Intervention and Outreach Network (VISION), was to leverage partnerships between healthcare providers, public health researchers, and concerned community stakeholders to promote secure firearm storage messaging and practices to prevent firearm suicides. The multidisciplinary VA team—which included an anthropologist, clinicians with suicide prevention expertise, and veterans—employed a multimethod approach to understand diverse community viewpoints, identify healthcare and community assets and resources for a public health intervention, and establish common language and goals to support sustainable partnerships (True et al. 2022). Ethnography was at the center of this work, both in informing formulation of the research goals and in building trust and establishing roles and relationships necessary to support implementation of interventions in community and clinical settings.

The genesis for this firearm suicide prevention research came from ethnographic work that Gala was conducting with a veteran and VA researcher (Ray Facundo) in Southeast Louisiana, using Photovoice methods to collaborate with post-9/11 veterans with traumatic brain injury and their families (Abraham et al. 2021; True et al. 2019; True et al. 2021; True et al. 2021; Wyse et al. 2020). In the course of that work, Gala and Ray spent time in the homes and community spaces of their collaborators and came to recognize the central role that firearms played in the lives of many Louisiana military families, as well as the number of veterans who had lost someone to firearm suicide or contemplated suicide by firearm themselves. At the same time, Gala was noticing the strong culture of gun shows in Louisiana, where billboards in her neighborhood advertised a monthly gun show and many families spent their weekends visiting the gun show together. Based on these observations and their connections with firearm-owning veterans and their families, Gala and Ray and several suicide prevention colleagues received funding for their next study, with the research goals and methods being informed by their community collaborators and several veteran partners included as advisors. This illustrates how having close knowledge of a community and the existing relationships that come from using ethnographic methods can lead to new research ideas and initiatives, with one project building onto the previous one and community collaborators remaining engaged across multiple studies.

Prior to obtaining research funding and in preparation for a proposal, Gala was curious about gun shows as settings for observational learning and to identify new partners, as well as a site for future suicide prevention interventions. She started going to gun shows on her own and mapping out the vendors who had tables, including categorizing the nature of each business and which vendors were regularly present across multiple shows. Over time, she began to approach some vendors who were firearm instructors or retailers to talk with them about VISION and learn what they thought about the issue of firearm suicide and suicide prevention. Many vendors were initially suspicious that she was trying to sell something or that VISION was a disguised attempt at "taking away people's guns," but they also had concerns about firearm suicide and a desire to help address the issue; as she showed up month after month, some of them began to trust Gala and vouch for her with others in the community. In this regard, Gala had very little power or credibility within the ethnographic space of the gun show. By building trusting relationships with a few key people, she was able to "borrow" their credibility to build additional connections. During this time, Gala did not carry a notebook at the gun show nor did she write down the names of people she spoke with; instead, she collected business cards when they were available and waited until she was alone in her car to write down recollections and impressions from her conversations and observations and to create an annotated map of vendors. While this was not an ideal means for recording data, it felt necessary given the belief circulating among some firearm owners that firearm-related research may be masking anti-gun efforts to track and control firearm ownership.

As someone who was neither a firearm owner nor a veteran, Gala recognized through these experiences the importance of having firearm owners and veterans as members of the research team, both for the credibility they could bring as cultural insiders when approaching potential community partners and the knowledge they could bring to documenting and analyzing interactions and observations (i.e., data). Thus, she and her VA colleagues included veterans who were firearm owners as paid members of the research team, called Veteran Peer Champions (VPCs), who could both help the researchers enter into new ethnographic spaces (e.g., gun shops) and participate in data collection events. VISION provided VPCs with a small stipend to compensate for their time and expertise and developed a shared memo that outlined the roles and responsibilities of VPCs and what support VPCs could expect from the VA research team. This written document, although simple and nonbinding, was important for establishing transparency and respect between collaborators and was helpful when a situation arose where a VPC was unable to uphold their role for personal reasons.

Another consideration in using ethnography as a key method for VISION centered on reflections about where "critical events" (in this case, conversations about the role of firearms in suicide and promoting secure firearm storage to prevent suicide) were taking place and were observable; namely, locations like gun shows, firearm retailers and ranges, gun clubs, and veterans service organizations (VSOs). As an anthropologist/folklorist, Gala suspected that success in engaging firearm owners and industry leaders (i.e., gun show vendors, firearm retailers, and instructors) in public health efforts to prevent firearm suicide lay in going to these potential partners in spaces where they were most comfortable and spending extended periods of time in those spaces. This allowed Gala and her research colleagues to learn the language, norms, and concerns of potential community collaborators. Many firearm owners, particularly leaders in firearm-owning communities, have norms about language that signal in-group/out-group status; for example, a person who uses the term "weapon" instead of "firearm" may be seen as biased against firearms, and it was important for Gala and colleagues to be aware of these norms.

Furthermore, when the research team left the healthcare setting to spend time in community spaces, this signaled respect for their community partners' time and positioned those partners as collaborators with essential knowledge and expertise. This in turn facilitated frank conversations where community members felt empowered to challenge and "test" the researchers early in the research process; this "testing" proved crucial for improving the researchers' ability to communicate effectively with new community contacts as the research moved forward. Gala's interactions with one key informant named John (a pseudonym) illustrate how this worked. When she first began to meet with John—a veteran who owned a prominent gun store and was well-connected in firearm-owning and veteran communities—she was introduced to John by a veteran who was employed as a member of the research team. At that initial meeting in his store, John was skeptical of Gala's intentions and believed the VA researchers were biased against firearms. As Gala visited his store multiple times, including coming on her own to spend time at the shooting range that was part of the store, John challenged her on the core premises of the research, including why suicide prevention research was focused on firearms rather than other suicide methods. Responding thoughtfully to John's questions prompted Gala and others on the research team to hone their messaging to preemptively address these concerns for future contacts. As a result, they developed a printed slide deck in PowerPoint consisting of answers to Frequently Asked Questions and infographics to explain and contextualize the focus on firearms in suicide prevention. These conversations between John and Gala, which could only have occurred in the context and across the timeline of ethnographic work, led to a foundation of trust and mutual respect such that John became one of the bigger champions of the research, serving as a connector to others in the firearm-owning community. In addition, John began to adopt the messaging that was created in response to his "testing"; in future meetings where a potential community collaborator voiced concerns or skepticism, John was often the one who stepped forward to explain the importance of focusing on firearms in suicide prevention. Like many key contacts in ethnographic work, John also had the potential to function as a "gatekeeper" who could potentially have blocked the researcher's access to some community members. John later shared with Gala that, had he not trusted her intentions or VISION's goals, he would have discouraged people he knew in the firearms community from collaborating. In this way, while using an ethnographic approach took more time than other methods, it also led to greater success in terms of gaining buy-in from key community partners, which then led to greater ability to connect with and gain the trust of additional collaborators.

As VISION evolved from Gala's solo explorations at gun shows to a multidisciplinary, team-based project across multiple ethnographic spaces, the importance of more formal training and procedures for conducting observations and conversations became apparent. To this end, the team held several in-person meetings for cross-training between the VA and community researchers. At these meetings, the VA investigators conducted education and training activities for the entire team based on their personal knowledge and expertise; for example, a psychologist and suicide prevention researcher shared key research findings on suicide among veterans and the role of secure firearm storage in suicide prevention. The veterans on the team trained the civilian researchers in "firearm cultural competency" by sharing preferred language around firearms (e.g., using "firearm" instead of "gun") and norms regarding firearm handling and storage during military service.

It was at one of these meetings that Ray suggested that each person on the team articulate and share in writing something about their positionality (who they were and what communities they identified with) and their "why" related to the research goals (why they cared about preventing firearm suicide and any personal experiences with the topic, if applicable). This process created opportunities for each team member to practice reflexivity and facilitated the development of personal connections and knowledge across team members. The resulting written product, each team member's "personal statement," was incorporated into the PowerPoint slide deck mentioned earlier so it could be shared with community collaborators, both to illustrate the team's diversity of perspectives and experiences and to encourage those partners to share their own views and history with regards to preventing firearm suicide.

These meetings served several important purposes, including: building trust and rapport between team members; facilitating and recognizing different types of knowledge and authority; further clarifying roles and responsibilities beyond what was delineated in the VPC memo; and setting the stage for how future team debriefing meetings would occur. The team discussed feasible and acceptable templates for structured and unstructured data collection, as well as procedures for identifying community contacts and ethnographic sites and attending data collection events together. In addition, the group decided it was important to start systematically documenting observations and conversations despite the risk of being seen as "tracking" by firearm owners. Gala was able to draft a structured fieldnote template (see Box 3.4) based on feedback from various research team members, as well as language that could be used to explain to community members why a researcher was taking notes (i.e., "we are taking written notes so we can remember important details of conversations, but we are not tracking any specific information about anyone's firearms or firearm ownership …"). It was also decided that, whenever possible, ethnographic observations and interviews would be conducted in pairs consisting of a VPC and a VA researcher.

As the person on the team with the most expertise in community-based ethnography, working with people from various disciplines who did not have familiarity with this approach, Gala was pushed by the others to create a very simple (1-page) and user-friendly template that reminded the note-taker of the project goals and specified what information was most important to record for each observation and conversation. Later, Gala set up an Excel spreadsheet where the content of all the templated notes could be extracted and organized by topic for data analysis and follow-up (e.g., which events and spaces might be opportunities for future data collection, which community contacts were potential partners to help pilot interventions based on findings from the ethnographic work, etc.).

Through this process, the team of four VA investigators and four VPCs successfully conducted over 80 ethnographic observations and interviews at a variety of gun shows, firearm retailers, gun clubs, and VSO meetings. Ongoing support of team members occurred in the form of quick debriefing meetings between researcher-VPC pairs after each data collection event and hour-long biweekly meetings with VPCs. Through these activities, Gala was able to discern when someone on the team needed additional support for themselves or a community contact; for example, many community partners disclosed previous experience with losing someone close to them to firearm suicide, so VISION added postvention resources to the information provided during introductory meetings with new partners. It increased trust in the project when a potential community partner expressed a need and the research team member was able to address that need immediately in the field.

Through the work described earlier, which had ethnographic methods and principles at its core, the VISION team developed the necessary relationships and community capacity to pilot and evaluate several interventions to promote secure firearm storage messaging and practices, including The Armory Project, a state-wide partnership with firearm retailers to raise awareness about the option of temporarily storing firearms outside the home and to provide voluntary out-of-home storage for firearm owners in need (Constans et al. 2023). As this intervention was being piloted, Gala and her colleagues heard about a major concern from firearm retailers who wanted to help prevent firearm suicide by providing out-of-home storage for firearm owners in need but were concerned about the possibility of being sued and losing their business in the event they returned someone's firearms and that person subsequently harmed themselves or someone else. A member of the research team, Matt Bailey, was a veteran with a legal and policy background; he and Gala were able to work with their firearm retailer partners to develop and pass state legislation that provided retailers who help someone in need with immunity from civil liability, provided they follow the law (Louisiana House Bill 260). This not only addressed a major barrier to a promising firearm suicide prevention intervention but also built trust that supported future firearm suicide prevention efforts in Louisiana by demonstrating that researchers cared about the needs and priorities of their community partners.

References

Abraham, Traci H., Sarah S. Ono, Helene Moriarty, Laraine Winter, Ryan E. Bender, Ray Facundo, and Gala True. 2021. "Revealing the Invisible Emotion Work of Caregivers: A Photovoice Exploration of Informal Care Provided by Family Caregivers for Post-9/11 Veterans with Traumatic Brain Injuries." *Journal of Head Trauma Rehabilitation* 36 (1): 25–33. https://doi.org/10.1097/HTR.0000000000000589.

Agar, Michael, and James MacDonald. 1995. "Focus Groups and Ethnography." *Human Organization* 54 (1): 78–86.

Aijazi, Omer, Emily Amburgey, Bina Limbu, Manoj Suji, James Binks, Courtney Balaz-Munn, Katharine Rankin, and Sara Shneiderman. 2021. "The Ethnography of Collaboration: Navigating Power Relationships in Joint Research." *Collaborative Anthropologies* 13 (2): 56–99. https://doi.org/10.1353/cla.2021.0003.

Bikker, Annemieke P., Helen Atherton, Heather Brant, Tania Porqueddu, John L. Campbell, Andy Gibson, Brian McKinstry, Chris Salisbury, and Sue Ziebland. 2017. "Conducting a Team-Based Multi-Sited Focused Ethnography in Primary Care." *BMC Medical Research Methodology* 17 (1): 139. https://doi.org/10.1186/s12874-017-0422-5.

Blackwell, Gretta. 2023. "Pursuing Ethnographic 'Closeness': A Reflection on Race, Reality Television Audiences, and the Focus Group Encounter." *Southern Communication Journal* 88 (5): 416–27. https://doi.org/10.1080/1041794X.2023.2232808.

Boland, Joshua, Susan Banks, Robin Krabbe, Suanne Lawrence, Therese Murray, Terese Henning, and Miriam Vandenberg. 2022. "A COVID-19-Era Rapid Review: Using Zoom and Skype for Qualitative Group Research." *Public Health Research & Practice* 32 (2): 31232112. https://doi.org/10.17061/phrp31232112.

Bond, Virginia, Fredrick Ngwenya, Emma Murray, Nothando Ngwenya, Lario Viljoen, Dumile Gumede, Chiti Bwalya, et al. 2019. "Value and Limitations of Broad Brush Surveys Used in Community-Randomized Trials in Southern Africa." *Qualitative Health Research* 29 (5): 700–718. https://doi.org/10.1177/1049732318809940.

Brunner, Julian, Melissa M. Farmer, Bevanne Bean-Mayberry, Catherine Chanfreau-Coffinier, Claire T. Than, Alison B. Hamilton, and Erin P. Finley. 2022. "Implementing Clinical Decision Support for Reducing Women Veterans' Cardiovascular Risk in VA: A Mixed-Method, Longitudinal Study of Context, Adaptation, and Uptake." *Frontiers in Health Services* 2 (September): 946802. https://doi.org/10.3389/frhs.2022.946802.

Bunce, Arwen E., Rachel Gold, James V. Davis, Carmit K. McMullen, Victoria Jaworski, MaryBeth Mercer, and Christine Nelson. 2014. "Ethnographic Process Evaluation in Primary Care: Explaining the Complexity of Implementation." *BMC Health Services Research* 14 (1): 607. https://doi.org/10.1186/s12913-014-0607-0.

Chazdon, Scott, Mary Emery, Debra Hansen, Lorie Higgins, and Rebecca Sero. 2017. "*A Field Guide to Ripple Effects Mapping*." University of Minnesota Libraries Publishing. https://conservancy.umn.edu/handle/11299/190639.

Closser, Svea, Anat Rosenthal, Kenneth Maes, Judith Justice, Kelly Cox, Patricia A. Omidian, Ismaila Zango Mohammed, Aminu Mohammed Dukku, Adam D. Koon, and Laetitia Nyirazinyoye. 2016. "The Global Context of Vaccine Refusal: Insights from a Systematic Comparative Ethnography of the Global Polio Eradication Initiative: Global Context of Vaccine Refusal." *Medical Anthropology Quarterly* 30 (3): 321–41. https://doi.org/10.1111/maq.12254.

Cohen, Amy N., Matthew J. Chinman, Alison B. Hamilton, Fiona Whelan, and Alexander S. Young. 2013. "Using Patient-Facing Kiosks to Support Quality Improvement at Mental Health Clinics." *Medical Care* 51 (March): S13–20. https://doi.org/10.1097/MLR.0b013e31827da859.

Constans, Joseph I., Claire Houtsma, Matthew Bailey, and Gala True. 2023. "The Armory Project: Partnering with Firearm Retailers to Promote and Provide Voluntary OUT-OF-HOME Firearm Storage." *Suicide and Life-Threatening Behavior* 53 (5): 716–24. https://doi.org/10.1111/sltb.12977.

DiCicco-Bloom, Barbara, and Benjamin F. Crabtree. 2006. "The Qualitative Research Interview." *Medical Education* 40 (4): 314–21. https://doi.org/10.1111/j.1365-2929.2006.02418.x.

Eaves, Emery R., Robert T. Trotter, Bonnie Marquez, Kayla Negron, Eck Doerry, David Mensah, Kate A. Compton-Gore, et al. 2022. "Possibilities and Constraints of Rapid Online Ethnography: Lessons from a Rapid Assessment of COVID-19 Policy for People Who Use Drugs." *Frontiers in Sociology* 7 (August): 959642. https://doi.org/10.3389/fsoc.2022.959642.

Emerson, Robert M., Rachel I. Fretz, and Linda L. Shaw. 2011. *Writing Ethnographic Fieldnotes*. 2nd ed. *Chicago Guides to Writing, Editing, and Publishing*. Chicago: The University of Chicago Press.

Fetters, Michael D., and Ellen B. Rubinstein. 2019. "The 3 Cs of Content, Context, and Concepts: A Practical Approach to Recording Unstructured Field Observations." *The Annals of Family Medicine* 17 (6): 554–60. https://doi.org/10.1370/afm.2453.

Finley, Erin P. 2011. *Fields of Combat: Understanding PTSD among Veterans of Iraq and Afghanistan*. Ithaca: ILR Press.

Finley, Erin P., Svea Closser, Malabika Sarker, and Alison B. Hamilton. 2023. "Editorial: The Theory and Pragmatics of Power and Relationships in Implementation." *Frontiers in Health Services* 3 (March): 1168559. https://doi.org/10.3389/frhs.2023.1168559.

Finley, Erin P., Sheila B. Frankfurt, Nipa Kamdar, David E. Goodrich, Elyse Ganss, Chien J. Chen, Christine Eickhoff, et al. 2024. "Partnership Building for Scale-up in the Veteran Sponsorship Initiative: Strategies for Harnessing Collaboration to Accelerate Impact in Suicide Prevention." *Health Services Research* 17 (1): 43. https://doi.org/10.1111/1475-6773.14309.

Finley, Erin P., Alexis K. Huynh, Melissa M. Farmer, Bevanne Bean-Mayberry, Tannaz Moin, Sabine M. Oishi, Jessica L. Moreau, et al. 2018. "Periodic Reflections: A Method of Guided Discussions for Documenting Implementation Phenomena." *BMC Medical Research Methodology* 18 (1): 153. https://doi.org/10.1186/s12874-018-0610-y.

Fix, Gemmae M., Bo Kim, Mollie A. Ruben, and Megan B. McCullough. 2022. "Direct Observation Methods: A Practical Guide for Health Researchers." *PEC Innovation* 1 (December): 100036. https://doi.org/10.1016/j.pecinn.2022.100036.

Gao, Yajing, Xuemei Chen, Wei Zhang, Qiuyi Wang, Jing Liu, and Lanshou Zhou. 2022. "Online Ethnography for People with Chronic Conditions: Scoping Review." *Journal of Medical Internet Research* 24 (11): e37941. https://doi.org/10.2196/37941.

Geertz, Clifford. 1973. "Thick Description: Toward an Interpretive Theory of Culture." In *The Interpretation of Cultures*, 310–23. Clifford Geertz, Editor. New York, New York: Basic Books.

Goedken, Cassie Cunningham, Daniel J. Livorsi, Michael Sauder, Mark W. Vander Weg, Emily E. Chasco, Nai-Chung Chang, Eli Perencevich, and Heather Schacht Reisinger. 2019. "'The Role as a Champion Is to Not Only Monitor but to Speak Out and to Educate':

The Contradictory Roles of Hand Hygiene Champions." *Implementation Science* 14 (1): 110. https://doi.org/10.1186/s13012-019-0943-x.

Greene, Jeremy A., Niteesh K. Choudhry, Elaine Kilabuk, and William H. Shrank. 2011. "Online Social Networking by Patients with Diabetes: A Qualitative Evaluation of Communication with Facebook." *Journal of General Internal Medicine* 26 (3): 287–92. https://doi.org/10.1007/s11606-010-1526-3.

Greenhalgh, Trisha, and Deborah Swinglehurst. 2011. "Studying Technology Use as Social Practice: The Untapped Potential of Ethnography." *BMC Medicine* 9 (1): 45. https://doi.org/10.1186/1741-7015-9-45.

Hamilton, Alison B., Melissa M. Farmer, Tannaz Moin, Erin P. Finley, Ariel J. Lang, Sabine M. Oishi, Alexis K. Huynh, Jessica Zuchowski, Sally G. Haskell, and Bevanne Bean-Mayberry. 2017. "Enhancing Mental and Physical Health of Women through Engagement and Retention (EMPOWER): A Protocol for a Program of Research." *Implementation Science* 12 (1): 23. https://doi.org/10.1186/s13012-017-0658-9.

Hamilton, Alison B., and Erin P. Finley. 2019. "Qualitative Methods in Implementation Research: An Introduction." *Psychiatry Research* 280 (October): 112516. https://doi.org/10.1016/j.psychres.2019.112516.

Hamilton, Alison B., Erin P. Finley, Bevanne Bean-Mayberry, Ariel Lang, Sally G. Haskell, Tannaz Moin, Melissa M. Farmer, and the EMPOWER QUERI Team. 2023. "Enhancing Mental and Physical Health of Women through Engagement and Retention (EMPOWER) 2.0 QUERI: Study Protocol for a Cluster-Randomized Hybrid Type 3 Effectiveness-Implementation Trial." *Implementation Science Communications* 4 (1): 23. https://doi.org/10.1186/s43058-022-00389-w.

Higginbottom, Gina, Jennifer Pillay, and Nana Boadu. 2015. "Guidance on Performing Focused Ethnographies with an Emphasis on Healthcare Research." *The Qualitative Report* 18 (17): 1–16. https://doi.org/10.46743/2160-3715/2013.1550.

Himmelman, Arthur T. 2002. "Collaboration for a Change: Definitions, Decision-Making Models, Roles, and Collaboration Process Guide." http://tennessee.edu/wp-content/uploads/2019/07/Himmelman-Collaboration-for-a-Change.pdf.

Kara, Hanna, Maija Jäppinen, Camilla Nordberg, and Anna-Leena Riitaoja. 2023. "The Ethical Performance of Access and Consent in Ethnographic Research on Social Work Encounters with Migrant-Background Service Users." *Qualitative Social Work* 22 (4): 663–78. https://doi.org/10.1177/14733250221088421.

Kornfield, Jack. 2009. *The Wise Heart: A Guide to the Universal Teachings of Buddhist Psychology*. New York: Bantam Books.

Lofland, John, and Lyn H. Lofland. 1995. *Analyzing Social Settings: A Guide to Qualitative Observation and Analysis*, 3rd ed. Belmont, CA: Wadsworth.

Maietta, Raymond, Paul Mihas, Kevin Swartout, Jeff Petruzzelli, and Alison Hamilton. 2021. "Sort and Sift, Think and Shift: Let the Data Be Your Guide an Applied Approach to Working With, Learning From, and Privileging Qualitative Data." *The Qualitative Report* 26 (6): 2045–60. https://doi.org/10.46743/2160-3715/2021.5013.

McGranahan, Carole. 2015. "What Is Ethnography? Teaching Ethnographic Sensibilities without Fieldwork." *Teaching Anthropology* 4: 23–36. (April). https://doi.org/10.22582/ta.v4i1.421.

McHugh, Siobhan, Laura Sheard, Jane O'Hara, and Rebecca Lawton. 2022. "The Feasibility and Acceptability of Implementing Video Reflexive Ethnography (VRE) as an Improvement Tool in Acute Maternity Services." *BMC Health Services Research* 22 (1): 1308. https://doi.org/10.1186/s12913-022-08713-9.

McInnes, D. Keith, Shawn Dunlap, Gemmae M. Fix, Marva V. Foster, Jennifer Conti, Jill S. Roncarati, and Justeen K. Hyde. 2022. "Longitudinal High-Frequency Ethnographic Interviewing to Simulate and Prepare for Intensive Smartphone Data Collection among Veterans with Homeless Experience." *Frontiers in Digital Health* 4 (August): 897288. https://doi.org/10.3389/fdgth.2022.897288.

Metz, Allison, Todd Jensen, Amanda Farley, Annette Boaz, Leah Bartley, and Melissa Villodas. 2022. "Building Trusting Relationships to Support Implementation: A Proposed Theoretical Model." *Frontiers in Health Services* 2 (September): 894599. https://doi.org/10.3389/frhs.2022.894599.

Monahan, Torin, and Jill A. Fisher. 2010. "Benefits of 'Observer Effects': Lessons from the Field." *Qualitative Research* 10 (3): 357–76. https://doi.org/10.1177/1468794110362874.

Neuwirth, Esther B., Jim Bellows, Ana H. Jackson, and Patricia M. Price. 2012. "How Kaiser Permanente Uses Video Ethnography of Patients for Quality Improvement, Such As in Shaping Better Care Transitions." *Health Affairs* 31 (6): 1244–50. https://doi.org/10.1377/hlthaff.2012.0134.

Palinkas, Lawrence A., and Douglas Zatzick. 2019. "Rapid Assessment Procedure Informed Clinical Ethnography (RAPICE) in Pragmatic Clinical Trials of Mental Health Services Implementation: Methods and Applied Case Study." *Administration and Policy in Mental Health and Mental Health Services Research* 46 (2): 255–70. https://doi.org/10.1007/s10488-018-0909-3.

Pilbeam, Caitlin, Trisha Greenhalgh, and Caroline M. Potter. 2023. "Ethnographic Closeness: Methodological Reflections on the Interplay of Engagement and Detachment in Immersive Ethnographic Research." *Journal of the Royal Anthropological Institute* 29 (4): 820–39. https://doi.org/10.1111/1467-9655.14007.

Pope, Catherine. 2005. "Conducting Ethnography in Medical Settings." *Medical Education* 39 (12): 1180–87. https://doi.org/10.1111/j.1365-2929.2005.02330.x.

Rankl, Felicia, Ginger A. Johnson, and Cecilia Vindrola-Padros. 2021. "Examining What We Know in Relation to How We Know It: A Team-Based Reflexivity Model for Rapid Qualitative Health Research." *Qualitative Health Research* 31 (7): 1358–70. https://doi.org/10.1177/1049732321998062.

Reisinger, Heather Schacht, John Fortney, and Greg Reger. 2021. "Rapid Ethnographic Assessment in Clinical Settings." In *Paths to the Future of Higher Education*, 117–34. Brian L. Foster, Steven W. Graham, and Joe F. Donaldson, Editors. Charlotte, NC: Information Age.

Richards, Helen, and Carol Emslie. 2000. "The 'doctor' or the 'Girl from the University'? Considering the Influence of Professional Roles on Qualitative Interviewing." *Family Practice* 17 (1): 71–75. https://doi.org/10.1093/fampra/17.1.71.

Sangaramoorthy, Thurka, and Karen A. Kroeger. 2020. *Rapid Ethnographic Assessments: A Practical Approach and Toolkit for Collaborative Community Research*. Abingdon, Oxon; New York, NY: Routledge, Taylor & Francis Group. https://doi.org/10.4324/9780429286650.

Shattuck, Daniel, Bonnie O. Richard, Elise Trott Jaramillo, Evelyn Byrd, and Cathleen E. Willging. 2022. "Power and Resistance in Schools: Implementing Institutional Change to Promote Health Equity for Sexual and Gender Minority Youth." *Frontiers in Health Services* 2 (November): 920790. https://doi.org/10.3389/frhs.2022.920790.

Stuckey, Heather L., Jennifer L. Kraschnewski, Michelle Miller-Day, Kimberly Palm, Caroline Larosa, and Christopher Sciamanna. 2014. "'Weighing' Two Qualitative Methods: Self-Report Interviews and Direct Observations of Participant Food Choices." *Field Methods* 26 (4): 343–61. https://doi.org/10.1177/1525822X14526543.

Tarrant, Carolyn, Barbara O'Donnell, Graham Martin, Julian Bion, Alison Hunter, and Kevin D. Rooney. 2016. "A Complex Endeavour: An Ethnographic Study of the Implementation of the Sepsis Six Clinical Care Bundle." *Implementation Science* 11 (1): 149. https://doi.org/10.1186/s13012-016-0518-z.

Taylor, Beck, Catherine Henshall, Sara Kenyon, Ian Litchfield, and Sheila Greenfield. 2018. "Can Rapid Approaches to Qualitative Analysis Deliver Timely, Valid Findings to Clinical Leaders? A Mixed Methods Study Comparing Rapid and Thematic Analysis." *BMJ Open* 8 (10): e019993. https://doi.org/10.1136/bmjopen-2017-019993.

True, Gala, Lawrence Davidson, Ray Facundo, David V. Meyer, Sharon Urbina, and Sarah S. Ono. 2021. "'Institutions Don't Hug People': A Roadmap for Building Trust, Connectedness, and Purpose through Photovoice Collaboration." *Journal of Humanistic Psychology* 61 (3): 365–404. https://doi.org/10.1177/0022167819853344.

True, Gala, Ray Facundo, Carlos Urbina, Sawyer Sheldon, J Duncan Southall, and Sarah Ono. 2021. "'If You Don't Name the Dragon, You Can't Begin to Slay It:' Participatory Action Research to Increase Awareness Around Military-Related Traumatic Brain Injury." *Journal of Community Engagement and Scholarship* 13 (4): 1–16. https://doi.org/10.54656/RUAU3402.

True, Gala, Amanda Raines, Ray Facundo, Matthew Bailey, Claire Houtsma, and Joseph J. Constans. 2022. "Community-Engagement and Coalition-Building to Promote Lethal Means Safety and Prevent Veteran Firearm Suicide." Poster presented at the National Research Conference on Firearm Injury Prevention, Washington, D.C., November.

True, Gala, Jessica Wyse, Laura Lorenz, Raymond Facundo, John Marmion, and Sarah Ono. 2019. "Therapeutic Effects of Participatory Action Research for Veterans and Caregivers Living With Brain Injury." *Archives of Physical Medicine and Rehabilitation* 100 (10): e135. https://doi.org/10.1016/j.apmr.2019.08.411.

Wolfinger, Nicholas H. 2002. "On Writing Fieldnotes: Collection Strategies and Background Expectancies." *Qualitative Research* 2 (1): 85–93. https://doi.org/10.1177/146879410200200l640.

Wyse, Jessica J., Sarah S. Ono, Margaret Kabat, and Gala True. 2020. "Supporting Family Caregivers of Veterans: Participant Perceptions of a Federally-Mandated Caregiver Support Program." *Healthcare* 8 (3): 100441. https://doi.org/10.1016/j.hjdsi.2020.100441.

CHAPTER 4

Ethnography for understanding

Analytic approaches

Selecting and applying analytic strategies and tools

As we discuss throughout the book, pragmatic healthcare ethnography can take many forms and can call upon a wide range of methods to address complex research questions. In Chapter 3, we describe commonly used methods such as observation and fieldnotes, ethnographic interviews, patient and provider interviews, focus groups, and periodic reflections. Qualitative analytic techniques can and will vary across these methods, depending on a number of factors, including pragmatic considerations such as timeline and resources.

In pragmatic healthcare ethnography, we emphasize analytic plans that have clear goals and strategies that are designed to address the research question(s). Several traditions in applied qualitative analysis inform the tools and strategies we describe in this chapter. For example, framework analysis, which has a strong history in applied research (Ritchie and Spencer 1994), is a good fit for studies with research objectives that are "clearly set and shaped by specific information requirements" and has been used in focused healthcare ethnographies (Ilott et al. 2016) and video ethnography (Lee and Bartlett 2021; Urquhart, Ker, and Rees 2018; Van Belle et al. 2020). Palinkas and Zatzick (2019), in their Rapid Assessment Procedure-Informed Clinical Ethnography (RAPICE) approach, describe "pragmatic data analysis" that can "incorporate different styles," including the tools that we describe later such as memos and codes. Similarly, in their ethnographic process evaluation in primary care, Bunce and colleagues (2014) note that "analysis of ethnographic data can take various forms," but is "essentially a dynamic process of organizing, describing, interpreting and legitimating raw (often text) data in order to make sense of the information."

We approach the process of selecting and applying analytic strategies and tools from the perspective of methodological pluralism. We do not advocate for any particular qualitative method paradigm (e.g., grounded theory) but rather for thinking about and through principles found across many paradigms. Of course, the more explicitly a project is tied to/grounded in a paradigm, the more aligned the analytic approach needs to be with that paradigm's principles (e.g., minimal or no use of deductive tools

DOI: 10.4324/9781003390657-4

in a phenomenological study), with proper citations and application of the relevant version(s) of that paradigm.

In this chapter, we describe ways to approach ethnographic data, select and use analytic tools, and move toward holistic understanding with those tools. We infuse this chapter with our suggestions for analysis *as conducted by a team*, since this is a key part of pragmatic healthcare ethnography (see Chapter 3). Another key focus is *thinking about analysis early (during study design!) and often*. For example, many steps taken by the data collection team will impact the nature of the data to be analyzed and the strategies available and accessible to the team. As we note in Chapter 3, consistency in data collection across the team is integral to efficiently moving through pragmatic ethnographic research. We wrap up the chapter by briefly reflecting on methodological rigor in qualitative data analysis, which has varying definitions, traditions, terminology, and components. In keeping with the theme of this book, we emphasize pragmatic applications of rigor, bearing in mind that our health- and healthcare-oriented ethnographic research is often mixed methods and may necessitate sharing language and concepts of rigor (e.g., replicability) that would not always be applicable nor valued in qualitative-only studies or in particular qualitative paradigms.

Approaching the data

Figure 4.1 depicts a general process for moving from research question(s) to study design (see Chapter 2), data collection (see Chapter 3), and data analysis, ultimately striving for holistic understanding. This chapter starts where Chapter 3 leaves off, with having data available and being ready to work with it, which does not necessarily mean having completed data collection. In pragmatic healthcare ethnography, data analysis should be concurrent with data collection depending on study design, need(s) for data, resources, and timeline. In fact, many of the "getting organized" tasks can begin prior to data collection, with an organizational system ready to populate when data become available. Later we walk through three steps toward approaching a body of ethnographic data for analysis: getting organized, getting familiar, and getting strategic (Figure 4.1).

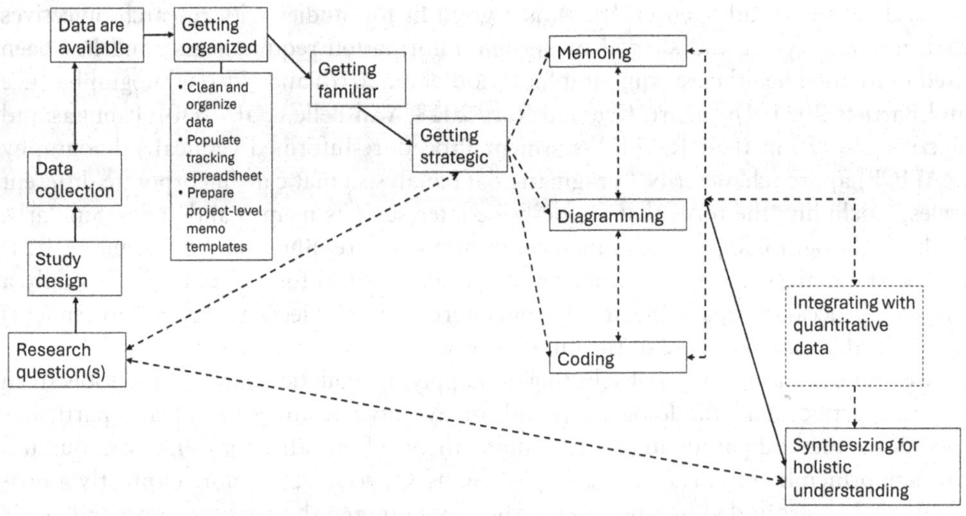

Figure 4.1 Moving from research question to data analysis and understanding

Getting organized

The organizational system for analysis should be an extension of the organizational system for data collection, which is necessary in a study of any size. With the multiple sources of data typical of ethnography, complexity is increased and usually requires knowledgeable and organized project managers. A more traditional free-form approach to processing the data can be challenging in a team-based environment because each analyst will follow their own line of thought without an explicit discussion and plan. While independent paths could yield interesting insights, the time and collective work it would take to reconcile multiple perspectives and pathways could far exceed the project's timeline and could perhaps result in a less than coherent analysis.

Organizing different sources of data—pulling together documents such as transcripts or fieldnotes—helps with pragmatically orienting toward next steps. The importance of good organization, particularly in pragmatic healthcare ethnography, should not be underestimated, as poor organization can derail timelines and group processes. Setting up and maintaining the organizational system is a consensus-based and dynamic team process. All involved need to have an understanding of and (authorized) access to sources of data and resources for analysis, such as specialized qualitative data analysis software. For example, in projects using transcripts, after "cleaning the data"—that is, checking and editing transcripts to ensure they have no transcription errors—a designated member of the team can create a "cleaned transcripts for analysis" folder.

A project spreadsheet tracking all data sources, when and where they were collected, who collected them, where they are located, who is working on them, and their status will serve as a go-to resource throughout the project. The spreadsheet needs to be continually populated and updated, preferably by one or two people working in close coordination. The spreadsheet (see Table 4.1) will likely evolve over time, as the need for different details arises and the team's procedures evolve. Finally, project-level memo templates (discussed later) can be set up and initiated (e.g., the methods memo can be populated with details about processes related to cleaning and storing transcripts).

Getting familiar

Deep familiarity with the ethnographic data is necessary for any analytic approach: we need to know what is in the data in order to think about how we are going to analyze it. Familiarization ideally begins during data collection, depending on whether the analyst is also involved in data collection. What we immediately "take home" from a data collection episode, such as an interview, will likely evolve as we collect more data. As data collection proceeds, we begin to reflect on that data within each episode and across episodes, for example by listening to interviews, reading transcripts, and reviewing fieldnotes. Because familiarity is so critical to ethnographic work, ideally at least some of the same team members should be involved from data collection, on through analysis, and into developing the end product(s).

Table 4.1 Example data spreadsheet

ID	*Interview complete*	*Transcript complete*	*Transcript cleaned*	*Summary complete*	*Analyst 1*	*Analyst 2*
MD7-102	Dec 5	Jan 2	Jan 9	Jan 20	AH	EF

There is no substitute for this first step of familiarization, which is central to most qualitative analytical approaches, although it may be achieved in different ways. Reading a subset (~3) of data sources (e.g., cleaned interview transcripts) can happen during an initial learning period (Maietta et al. 2021). Those on the analysis team can independently read and come together to share reflections ideally documented in memos (see later). We encourage getting to know the data thoroughly before deciding which tools to use first, as the data will inform decisions about ways of capturing and synthesizing information, as we will explain further.

Getting strategic

As we get familiar with what is in the data, we can begin to think about analytic tools that will be a good initial "fit" with the data. Ethnographies typically draw upon multiple methods or data sources, as we describe in Chapters 2 and 3, and thus may necessitate multiple analytic tools, as well as different tools at different times, for different purposes. Flexibility and openness to trying different tools, even if they were not specified before the study, are essential for letting the "data be your guide" (Maietta et al. 2021).

Qualitative data sources can be considered on a spectrum from unstructured to structured data (Figure 4.2). Unstructured data, such as extemporaneous fieldnotes or unstructured interviews, may be most amenable to free-form memoing and diagramming, to begin processing quotations, key ideas, questions, observations, and directions. Unstructured data collection, while valuable, is challenging in a pragmatic context. As we note throughout the book, having at least some semi-structured elements of data collection in pragmatic healthcare ethnography can be helpful for team-based work (including analysis) and moving to products on a specific timeline. Semi-structured data is also amenable to rapid qualitative analysis, which can further help with completing focused analyses on a tight timeline (Hamilton and Finley 2019). Rapid qualitative analysis involves more structured memoing in the form of templated summaries that are organized by key domains from the data collection instruments. This rapid analytic approach is not a good fit for unstructured data (Taylor et al. 2018). The key consideration we are emphasizing here is that *strong alignment between data collection instruments and analytic tools will enhance a pragmatic approach to analysis.*

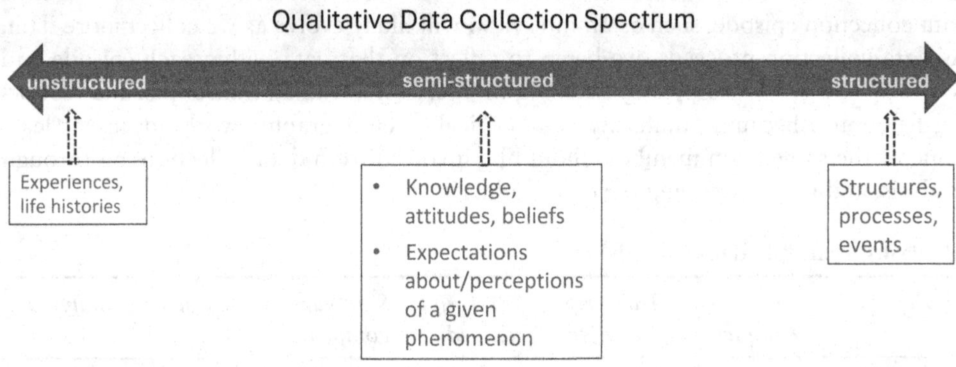

Figure 4.2 Qualitative data collection spectrum

Later we discuss using three analytic processes—memoing, diagramming, and coding—that yield the analytic tools of memos, diagrams, and codes. These are not the only analytic tools available to qualitative researchers, but we find that they are our go-to tools in pragmatic ethnographic team-based analysis.

Using tools: Memoing

In our experience, one analytic process—memoing—works well and is in fact essential for analysis of different types of qualitative data (Maietta et al. 2021). Memos are an important space for reflexive writing, capturing nascent and evolving interpretations, emergent questions, thoughts, next steps, and personal "jottings" (emotions, experiences), and can be an important tool *during* ethnographic data collection as well. These memos should be kept separate from fieldnotes. Fieldnotes are meant to serve as a source of data, wherein the researcher documents observations during the time(s) of data collection.

As an analytic tool, we recommend four types of project memos as essential (methods, research questions, emergent discoveries, and future studies) and two as optional but very helpful (episode profiles and topic memos) (see Table 4.2). The first four memo types can be set up while getting organized or at any point in the project (Maietta et al. 2021). Episode profiles and topic memos can be used any time after data collection has begun to support analytic thinking. All of these memos serve as evolving, cumulative resources. We suggest these labels for the different types of memos, but labels can be modified to suit a team's or project's needs.

Methods memos

Methods memos document all steps that are taken methodologically throughout analysis, or even from the beginning of the study. These memos can have a minimal structure, with sections for each phase of the project. For example, if changes are made to a data collection instrument (interview guide, observation template, etc.) during a data collection phase, these changes should be documented, with the date and reason for the changes.

Table 4.2 Common types of memos in pragmatic analysis

Memo type	*Purpose*
Methods	■ Documents key steps in data collection and analysis, including changes to methods or staff ■ Helpful if team members leave or join project ■ Can aid in developing methods sections of products
Research questions	■ Usually one per research question ■ Summarizes relevant lessons and key data sources
Emergent discoveries	■ Document novel lessons ("aha" moments) emerging across data sources
Future research	■ Ideas for later projects
Episode profile	■ Brief summary or reflection on a data collection event (e.g., interview)
Topic	■ Brings together key information on a specific topic from across data sources

In pragmatic ethnographic analysis, we create a separate methods memo for each type of data being collected in the project (e.g., Focus Group Methods Memo). Changes to the team should also be documented, with dates and any shifts in roles and responsibilities. During analysis, the methods memos should describe each step and decision in the analytic process. The methods memos should be detailed and thorough, lending to transparency of description (e.g., in methods sections of manuscripts) and rigor, as discussed further later.

Research question memo

Particularly in pragmatic healthcare ethnography, we recommend creating a memo for each research question throughout analysis. We usually have one memo per research question. In this memo, we write about what we are learning related to that question, with specific reference to where the learning came from (e.g., reading transcript [x], reviewing fieldnotes from [date]) and how the learning pertains to the research question. As with other memoing, writing about what is being learned does not have to be formal or perfectly articulated; it just needs to be intelligible and useful. A memo for each research question becomes a go-to resource, for example, if a constituent asks what is emerging about a question they have posed, the analyst can go to this memo and at least begin to prepare a summary, likely with some reference back to raw data to add detail and nuance to the response (Maietta et al. 2021). In a study examining implementation of a new case management intervention for veterans experiencing homelessness, we might focus a research question memo specifically on veterans' perspectives on their case management experiences. In addition to providing an opportunity to develop a deeper understanding of this "slice" of the data, such memos can later be helpful in integrating perspectives toward a more holistic understanding of the dataset as a whole.

Emergent discoveries memo

Throughout analysis (and likely data collection as well), it is highly likely that we will discover things that we did not know before we started collecting and analyzing data. While these discoveries should be captured throughout several data collection tools, we have found it handy to have an emergent discoveries memo. This memo can serve as one place where all of the insightful, "aha" moments can be documented, cross-referencing other analytic tools where these moments may be more fully articulated. In Alison's emergent discoveries memo in her ethnographic study of women and methamphetamine use, she noted, "I had no idea that women's relationships with their mothers would be so salient to their substance use," and, "It didn't occur to me until the first interview that women were not only victims of violence, but also some were perpetrators. This changed my whole way of asking about violence, and I have to think about this and learn more."

Future studies memo

Inevitably, during data collection and analysis, we think of other studies that we want to do in the future. Jotting these ideas down in a future studies memo can be helpful for capturing new project ideas.

Episode profiles

Other types of memoing may or may not be employed in a given analysis. We make consistent use of *episode profiles* in our own work (Maietta et al. 2021). This type of memo can be unstructured and extemporaneous, developed for example while reading a transcript. The memo in Box 4.1 is an example from Alison's ethnographic work with women who were in residential treatment for methamphetamine use. An unstructured approach to this type of memo would be a good fit with unstructured data, such as life history interviews. In the memo excerpt shown in Figure 4.3, Alison was reflecting on the context of initiation and continuation of substance use and included musings about the notion of "functioning." This memo and a memo for each participant's story were Alison's way of processing thoughts and questions as she made her way through the data. They contain emergent questions (which could also be consolidated across documents in a project-level memo) as well as several direct quotes, in order to stay "grounded" in the data. Through this process of memoing about each person's narrative in relation to core topics, and layering in additional analytic work from tools described later, patterns began to crystallize into key findings, such as different patterns of methamphetamine use initiation among young Latinas and implications for intervention. This is one example of how memos can be not only an important analytic step toward answering core research questions, as noted earlier, but can also give rise to additional findings and products. This latter analysis was later published in a special issue of the *Journal of Ethnicity in Substance Abuse* on urban ethnography (Cheney et al. 2018).

With semi-structured and structured qualitative data, episode profiles can take a more structured form. In rapid qualitative analysis, a structured approach to the episode profile draws upon key domains (or "index categories;" Ritchie and Spencer 1994) in the data collection instrument (e.g., structured field note template, semi-structured interview guide) to design a template for summarizing the data (Hamilton and Finley 2019; St. George et al. 2023). Individual templated summaries are then created for each data collection

Box 4.1 Sample episode profile (partial)

Maria went from drinking to coke to speed to glass as of age 14. She attributes the initiation of drug use to either being molested when she was younger or to the loss of her sister-in-law—she can't "pinpoint where exactly." Another friend experienced a loss too, so they started drinking together, "just not to feel." I'm really interested in this idea of numbing feelings. She says she was partying a lot and didn't finish high school. She also says she started doing crystal to lose weight, that she was "doing it undercover" at her house. Her self-esteem was low, and she wanted to "sit in a crowd." Her parents didn't notice what she was up to. She did work and used coke to stay awake—she got it from the people she worked with. Because some of my participants have talked about using speed to function/work, I asked her if she was able to keep her job, and she said no, that she was a "dysfunctional addict." There does seem to be a popular notion among these women that there are functional and dysfunctional addicts—some that can keep going while using, and some that can't. What always intrigues, especially with those who can't keep working, is how do they afford their habits? I asked Maria this question and she said that she slept around, hustled, did "what she had to do"—lie, steal, cheat....

episode; these are valuable in and of themselves because they serve as a handy, at-a-glance guide to what is in the data, including snippets of direct quotations and cross-references to the raw data. We use the summaries for many purposes, including to inform each wave of data collection in longitudinal studies and to orient new team members to the dataset. For example, a new team member can listen to recorded interviews (this also helps with orienting to data collection techniques on the team), read transcripts, and review associated summaries in order to get familiar with the data and learn the technique of moving from raw data to summaries. In later analyses, summaries can be used in conjunction with other tools like matrices, which pull topic domains from the summaries into tables, thus providing a different view of the data, compiled across the sample (or by subsample). Furthermore, summaries can inform the development of other tools, such as topic memos and codes, as described later. It is important to note that with more structured analytic approaches like these, it is essential to maintain space for discovery (what lies beyond the structure) and not use the structure as a crutch or substitute for deep engagement with the data. In our summary templates, we have space at the end for "important quotations" and for "other observations," that is, material that does not fit within the set domains but is important to document in an "at-a-glance" overview of the data collection episode.

Variations on structured episode profiles abound (Lewinski et al. 2021; Nevedal et al. 2021). Alison and Erin and their teams keep the summaries closely aligned with what is in the data and document reflections about the data collection episodes in separate memos. Gemmae also prepares structured episode profiles for all data collection activities, jotting linear notes during data collection on a notepad or in the interview guide. As soon as possible—ideally immediately after data collection—she writes three main takeaways at the top of the document. Regardless of the approach used (i.e., with or without reflective/interpretive content), these memos serve as invaluable resources to quickly "recall" each data collection episode.

Topic memos

Topic memos can also be valuable tools during analysis. Topic memos may or may not correspond to discrete research questions, domains in data collection instruments, and/or codes (see later). They typically cut across data collection episodes, that is, they bring together what is being learned about a given topic across data, such as from interviews and observations. In topic memos, we recommend documenting where the topic came from/originated, why the topic is important (which could evolve over time), and what is being learned about the topic. In Alison's methamphetamine study, she developed memos related to several topics, for example, using meth for the first time, "numbing" feelings, "functioning" as an "addict," "affording my habit," and perpetrating violence. Note that some of these topics were labeled with the words of the participants, which helps with staying close to and being reminded of the data. These topic memos gave Alison an opportunity to document ideas and observations in an ongoing fashion as she reviewed transcripts of these unstructured, in-depth interviews. Topic memos serve as a resource to return to (or to "mine"; Maietta et al. 2024) frequently as opportunities for further analysis and dissemination arise. For example, Alison prepared a conference presentation on emotions, the brain, and methamphetamine, using both narrative data from the interviews and neurological research. In other words, analytically, content from a topic memo could be reviewed and reported on, and it could also be layered with other analytic resources (e.g., codes) to develop products.

Using tools: Diagramming, visual displays, and analytic templates

Ethnographic data can take many visual as well as textual forms. In turn, analysis of ethnographic data can be supported by the use of visual displays, such as diagrams. Diagrams may be used in ethnographic fieldnotes to depict settings, movement, relationships (e.g., relational diagrams such as kinship charts), processes, and histories. For example, as we note in Chapter 3, Alison and colleagues mapped out space in outpatient mental health clinics as they were introducing kiosks where patients could sit and input their symptoms and concerns. Analytically, these maps (or diagrams) can be explored and synthesized, perhaps along with interview data and/or other types of data, to describe how physical settings and objects affect (and are affected by) healthcare services.

In Alison's methamphetamine study, as she was engaging in analysis by reading transcripts, she began by creating a table with some key points of demographic and life history information (Table 4.3). While this was useful and became an important resource throughout the analysis, it was insufficient for capturing the complex timeline of each person's life and the description of her experiences along that timeline. Alison began drawing a timeline of each participant's life as shared by the participant in the interview and in a background survey, noting key junctures such as substance use starts and shifts (e.g., changes in substances used, changes in ways of using), sexual experiences, experiences of violence, pregnancies and pregnancy-related experiences (e.g., abortion, miscarriage, birth), educational transitions (e.g., dropping out of school), and treatment experiences (e.g., residential treatment). Creating this diagram for each person allowed Alison to discern patterns and shifts within and across each participant's narrative. The diagrams also served as a constant resource for different types of analyses, geared toward different types of products.

For a poster for a health-related conference (The College on Problems of Drug Dependence), Alison explored the relationship between child sexual abuse and methamphetamine use. Her analysis involved comparing and contrasting the diagrams of 13 women who described histories of child sexual abuse. Alison selected three for a poster, "Life trajectories of women methamphetamine users with child sexual abuse histories" (Figure 4.3). While all of the diagrams were interesting, Alison decided to feature trajectories of narratives from women of different ages and ethnicities. She used shading to indicate age at first use of methamphetamine, and included quotations from each woman's interview, pertaining to her first use of substances. For this analysis, these diagrams served as both a powerful analytic tool and a visual means for sharing the findings (as we address further in Chapter 5). For a chapter in an anthropology-related edited volume (Hamilton 2012), Alison focused analytically on women's experiences of pregnancy, creating spin-off diagrams focused solely on periods of pregnancy and exploring relationship issues, health, and methamphetamine and other substance use during and surrounding pregnancy. This analysis took a theoretical direction as Alison was

Table 4.3 Sample brief summary of life history information

Age	*Ethnicity*	*Highest education*	*# Children*	*First child at?*	*First started using?*	*Who introduced?*	*Sexual activity w/meth*	*Violence w/meth*	*First sexual experience*	*Trauma history*

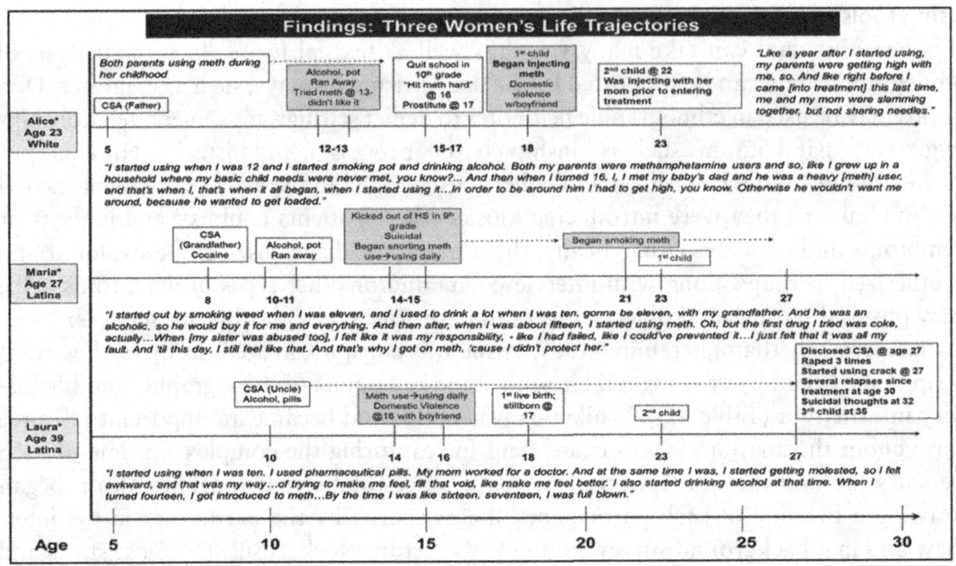

Figure 4.3 Sample diagram of life history trajectories (Hamilton and Goeders 2010)

interested in a theory (called "vital conjunctures"; Johnson-Hanks 2002) that offered a way to explore the data around a highly salient life experience.

In the case study from Heather Reisinger accompanying Chapter 1, the team used workflow maps to summarize clinic-level processes and invite feedback and collaborative planning from local teams. Together, these examples convey that *our analytic tools (such as diagrams) may serve many purposes, providing opportunities for discovery and evidence for different types of products*.

Finally, in an example of how diagramming can be used as part of a mixed-methods analysis, Brunner and colleagues (2022), including Erin and Alison, drew upon periodic reflections data (see Chapter 3) to create "timeline maps" summarizing contextual features and implementation efforts at each site, as part of an analysis of factors associated with successful adoption of a novel cardiovascular risk reduction template into the electronic medical record in five VA sites. They reviewed the reflections data for each site to develop a preliminary timeline map, then shared these with the implementation team to provide an opportunity for member checking, inviting corrections, and additional information about how the team engaged with each site. After the contextual factors and strategies used at each site were agreed upon, they then added quantitative findings to the timeline maps to create mixed-methods joint displays (Guetterman, Fetters, and Creswell 2015), demonstrating how contextual events and team activities were temporally associated with use of the template in each clinic. Again, the visual timeline approach offered an analytic process for working through the qualitative data to be able to "see" patterns (and anomalies) that pertained to the research question, and in this case, to integrate relevant quantitative data to explore adaptive approaches to implementation. Ultimately, the maps also served as a product for illustrating the results in a publication (Figure 4.4).

In the Sort and Sift, Think and Shift method (Maietta et al. 2024), diagramming may include using shapes in Microsoft PowerPoint to bring quotations or other segments of

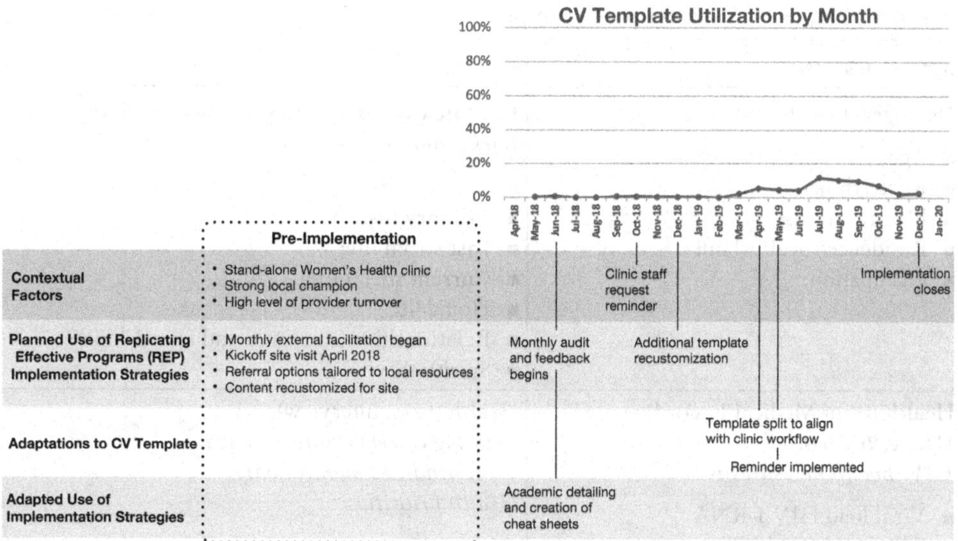

Figure 4.4 Sample "timeline map" for visualizing mixed-method data (Reproduced with permission from Brunner et al. 2022)

data together, shift them, explore meanings and connections, create categories, and follow hunches. This approach can be used with unstructured and semi-structured qualitative data and with many types of data, including fieldnotes, transcripts, documents, etc. This process dovetails well with mixed-methods analytic techniques, for example, quantitative results can be added to the diagrams to begin to visualize possible connections.

Teams conducting pragmatic ethnography can use other available software to organize data, such as Excel, Word, or PowerPoint programs in the Microsoft Office Suite or their Google analogs Sheets, Docs, or Slides (Meyer and Avery 2009). These programs are often ubiquitous in contemporary workplaces, making data analysis easier across distributed team members. Team members might not all have access to or skills for specialized qualitative data analysis software, but are likely to have access to and familiarity with more ubiquitous programs.

Microsoft Excel or Google Sheets are best used when data is fixed, relatively straightforward (not conceptual or theoretical), and amenable to being put in fixed rows and columns. Similarly, Gemmae has frequently employed analytic templates in Word to systematically catalog data. She has found this approach useful given that many of her projects involve team members at different locations who do not have access to the same specialized software. Similar to what Alison did in her methamphetamine and women project (see Table 4.3), for an ethnography comprising interviews, observation, and medical record review of people aging with HIV, Gemmae developed an analytic synthesis template to summarize all of the key data points for each participant in one place. The template included topics raised by the participants during their interviews, including trauma, past and current social activities, home life, and their descriptions of health priorities (see Table 4.4). Medical record data about HIV status, active medications, and comorbidities were also collected and added to the patient templates. The research question was focused on patients' experiences of aging with HIV in the context of their overall clinical health and social context.

Table 4.4 Sample analytic synthesis template

<table>
<tr><th>Key clinical issue</th><th>Key life issue</th></tr>
<tr><td>Demographics (from Survey)
■ Age:
■ Race/ethnicity:
■ Marital status:
■ Residence/rural/urban:
■ Occupation:</td><td>Key Life Context (from Interview)
Background/early life:
■ Past traumas:
■ Military history:
■ Past social life:
■ Current social life:
■ Home life:
■ Relationships (romantic and friendships):
■ Spirituality:</td></tr>
<tr><td>Health (from Medical Record)
Date extracted.
HIV (health measures):
■ Viral load HIV-1 RNA
■ WBC (AUTOMATED)
■ CD3+/CD4+ #
■ EGFR
■ SGPT/ATL
■ SGOT/AST
■ BMI
■ Hemoglobin
Active Medications:
Comorbidities:</td><td rowspan="2">Health (from interview)
Framing of HIV [note absence]:
Comorbidities mentioned:
Health priorities:</td></tr>
<tr><td>Health Related Quality of Life (Survey)
■ Mental Function Score:
■ Physical Function Score:
■ HIV Quality of Life Score:</td></tr>
<tr><td rowspan="4">Medical Record Data
(information recorded in notes):</td><td>Patient Reported Health Behaviors
(from interview)
■ Diet, activities, and management strategies:
■ Providers
■ Treatment (Rx?)
■ Health History/Context:</td></tr>
<tr><td>Illness beliefs (from interview)
■ Experience with HIV:
■ Acquisition/Cause:
■ Health Beliefs
■ Relationship between conditions:</td></tr>
<tr><td>Other/Social Determinants:
■ Finance/SES:
■ Politics</td></tr>
<tr><td>Intervention Ideas/Primary Needs:</td></tr>
</table>

Once the data were organized into the templates, Gemmae began sorting through the templates looking for patterns. She noted variation in how patients talked about their lives and what elements they emphasized as important. As a second analytic step, Gemmae used an approach similar to the Sort and Sift method described earlier. During a team meeting, they discussed how two participants had siblings who were murdered at a young age, a strikingly traumatic event. One participant surprisingly marked the event as something that happened in the past ("It was a long time ago, so if I sound cavalier about it, I'm not."). Through further team discussion about why this significant event might be described in such banal terms, the team began thinking about the concept of temporality. The resulting paper described three patterns of temporal orientation (Figures 4.5–4.7), with concomitant approaches to health management: past, present, and future-focused (Fix et al. 2021). This is also an example of how pragmatic ethnography can contribute to theory development, in this case why patients who might clinically look similar have different approaches to managing their health. These three temporal orientations were later used by Gemmae and her team to create sample patient composites, which have been used in two follow-up studies as an interview prompt. These cases feel authentic to providers being interviewed because they are based on patients' lived experience. The composite patients provide an opportunity for clinicians to discuss strategies for managing their own complex patients.

Using tools: Coding

Coding as an analytic tool is helpful when we are seeking understanding across a dataset. It entails a process of: identifying cross-cutting topics, ideas, or potential themes; creating and applying labels for those topics to relevant segments of text (or other forms of data); and reviewing and combining the topics to better understand what meaning-making is occurring across the data. *We caution against rushing to code, and do not recommend coding before at least getting familiar with the data.* Without a thorough understanding of each data collection episode, much time can be spent creating and

Ernest

68 years old; single, Black male.

Lives alone. "Retired" with many part-time jobs.

Active Problems (N=15; obesity, osteoarthrosis, PTSD, major depressive disorder, cocaine abuse)

Active Medications N=12

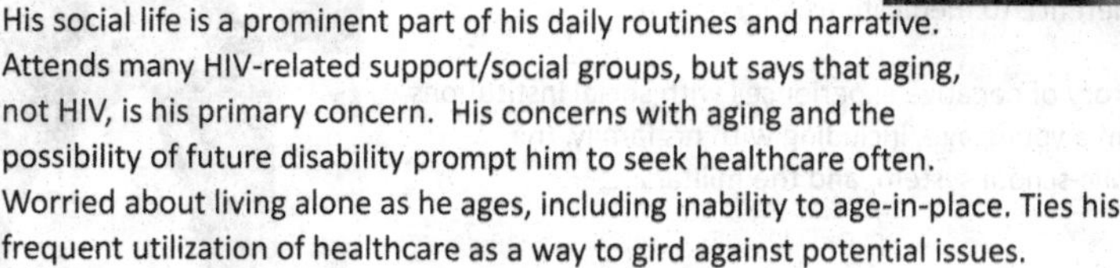

His social life is a prominent part of his daily routines and narrative.
Attends many HIV-related support/social groups, but says that aging, not HIV, is his primary concern. His concerns with aging and the possibility of future disability prompt him to seek healthcare often.
Worried about living alone as he ages, including inability to age-in-place. Ties his frequent utilization of healthcare as a way to gird against potential issues.

Figure 4.5 Sample composites summarizing distinct features of patient experience—Ernest

Source: Figure Photo 1, "Ernest" https://commons.wikimedia.org/wiki/File:Black_bearded_man_smiling,_2442565.jpg Leroy Skalstad, CC0, via Wikimedia Commons Attribution not legally required

Daniel
60 years old; single, white male.
Active Problems (N=18, including HIV, tobacco use, bipolar disorder, history of alcoholism, agoraphobia)
Active Medications (N= 13)

Poor medication adherence.

Not working. Lives alone, lonely & isolated.
Few family or social connections. 1 of 7 siblings, but estranged from much of his large, Irish family. He ties his drinking to lost family connections, never marrying or having children. However, rather than just improving his health, sobriety resulted in diminished social relationships. He laments his current state of loneliness.

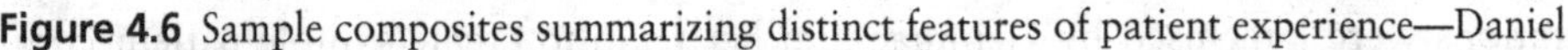

Figure 4.6 Sample composites summarizing distinct features of patient experience—Daniel

Source: FigurePhoto2, "Daniel" https://commons.wikimedia.org/wiki/File:Homeless_man_in_Milwaukee,_Wisconsin_-_2009.tiff Leroy Allen Skalstad, Public domain, via Wikimedia Commons

applying codes that ultimately do not serve the analysis. Pragmatically, this would not be a good use of an analyst's time.

Alison and her colleagues (Maietta et al. 2024) refer to coding as "topic monitoring," which speaks to the process of identifying and observing what happens with topics—and combinations of topics—as we work with the data. Coding is often misunderstood as synonymous with qualitative analysis, or the idea that once data are available, they are coded, and if coding has not been done, the data were not analyzed (or were not analyzed appropriately/thoroughly). On the contrary, *all work with the qualitative data is analysis, and robust analyses can be done without coding* (e.g., by memoing and/or diagramming). In analyzing data from ethnographic studies, we have found that coding can be useful, but is not always necessary in order to move to synthesizing for understanding.

Carl
61 years old; single, Black male.
History of homelessness; currently living in a rented room.

Active Problems (N= 14, including HIV, HCV, inactive TB)
Active Rx (N=11)

Mistrust of providers' recommendation and poor adherence to medications.

History of negative experiences with social institutions from a young age, including with his family, the public-school system, and the military.

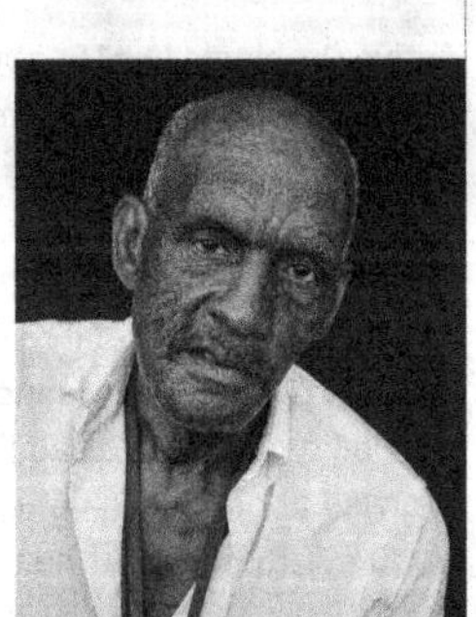

Figure 4.7 Sample composites summarizing distinct features of patient experience—Carl

Source: Figure Photo 3, "Carl" https://commons.wikimedia.org/wiki/File:Portrait_of_an_old_black_man,_BW.jpg Leroy Skalstad, CC0, via Wikimedia Commons

Here we review the approaches to coding that have worked on our analysis teams, with a few key premises: (1) coding should never precede data familiarization and is rarely the first step once data become available; (2) coding should not be done just to appease reviewers or others external to the team; (3) coding should have a cross-cutting purpose (i.e., used to connect data sources in order to discern meaning); and (4) coding should not be done in isolation without other tools that support contextualization, such as memos.

In our projects, typically an extensive amount of work has been done with the data prior to coding, if coding happens at all. For example, transcripts have been reviewed and perhaps memos and/or diagrams have been developed. These processes alone may be sufficient for several types of products that are generated in pragmatic healthcare ethnography (see Chapter 5). However, for ease of access to cross-cutting topics—whether *a priori* or emergent—codes may be useful, particularly in studies with large sample sizes, multiple sites, multiple waves of data collection, and/or multiple types of data, including quantitative data. Initially, codes may be derived from key topics that were intentionally and explicitly explored in the data collection efforts (e.g., the ethnographic interviews); these would be considered *deductive* codes and will likely be replete with data because data collection focused on these topics.

Our teams often engage in the application of these deductive codes, sometimes referred to as "top-down" or "high-level" coding. For example, in Alison's study of implementing an evidence-based treatment for methamphetamine, Alison initially applied the code "attitudes toward manualized treatment"; this code was applied to all instances in which participants expressed these attitudes. Consistent with a "template" approach to analysis (Crabtree and Miller, 1999; Brooks et al. 2015; King 2012), this type of coding can be useful to pull data together into different "buckets" that are known to the researcher to be important to the goals of the study. Codes are most useful when they have adequate data in them (Morse 2017); reviewing code "output" (i.e., the data to which the code has been applied) is an important step in assessing how useful the code will be (and how it will be useful) and deciding whether it needs to be broken down into component concepts, or perhaps merged with other codes to create a more robust concept with more evidence. In the case of the "attitudes toward manualized treatment" code, Alison eventually needed to parse out these attitudes as she began to understand a spectrum of attitudes that differed across researchers and practitioners. As noted earlier, deductive codes may be complemented by topic memos (e.g., Alison also developed an "attitudes toward manualized treatment" memo) that provide a space for writing about what is being learned as data are reviewed and codes are applied.

Relying on deductive, *a priori* coding alone may be sufficient for some purposes, for example, descriptive reports about particular topics or combinations of topics. However, we typically find that eventually, additional codes are needed to capture what is being identified in and learned from the data that was not necessarily anticipated. These codes would be considered *inductive* or *emic* codes (Morse 2017). In our pragmatic work, we often arrive at a hybrid approach to coding, with a combination of deductive and inductive codes. Fereday and Muir-Cochrane (2006) offer a detailed account of this hybrid approach in the analysis of qualitative data, and Proudfoot (2023) describes how a hybrid approach integrates with quantitative methods. A frequent challenge is moving beyond descriptions of the code content, to "themes," or expressions that are conceptually linked (Ryan and Bernard 2003), which may be founded in repetition of concepts, metaphors, similarities and differences in expressions, and other patterns (including absence of information) across the data.

To continue the example earlier, "attitudes toward manualized treatment" is not a theme—it is a topic that Alison monitored. Within that topic, Alison identified a theme among practitioners of a sense of loss of clinical intuition and creativity in the context of manualized treatment (Obert et al. 2005). This theme had important implications for how to train and support practitioners in the delivery of manualized treatment.

When we turn to coding as an analytic approach, we typically do so with the support of qualitative data analysis software. Such software provides sophisticated data management tools that are well-suited to larger and more complex studies (e.g., studies with multiple sites, types of participants, waves of data collection). Notably, the other tools and approaches (e.g., rapid qualitative analysis) we discuss in this chapter do not require specialized software. The use of specialized software should be intentional, as it requires knowledge, skills, and funds and may not be necessary to achieve the goals of a pragmatic ethnographic project.

Synthesizing for holistic understanding

In ethnographic studies, the goal is not only to analyze each dataset within the ethnography but to layer and integrate findings across datasets in order to achieve a holistic understanding. This layering and integrating process may necessitate revisiting the initial research goals or questions and re-engaging some methods along the way (e.g., conducting additional interviews or more observation) as new questions emerge. It may also entail integrating qualitative and quantitative data in a mixed-methods fashion (Fetters, Curry, and Creswell 2013; Miller et al. 2013). In Heather's case study (see Chapter 1), we learn about her process of conducting interviews, taking notes, debriefing, and sketching out maps, all of which resulted in the compilation of clinical workflow maps that themselves became vehicles for discussion and holistic understanding. In her case study (see Chapter 2), Megan described layering multiple sources of data to understand the roles of clinical pharmacy practitioners. Integration of multiple sources of data is challenging and potentially time-consuming, and is greatly aided by consistent and intentional organization of each dataset's details as well as points of potential convergence and expansion across the datasets (Palinkas 2014; Palinkas, Mendon, and Hamilton 2019).

Conclusion: Rigorous pragmatic ethnography

Now that we have described ethnographic study design, methods for pragmatic healthcare ethnography, and analytic approaches, let's return to Greenhalgh and Swinglehurst's (2011) criteria for evaluating the rigor of ethnography in terms of: (1) how successfully the ethnographic team achieves *authentic* immersion in the setting; (2) how *plausible* are the explanations achieved about the relevant phenomena, and the degree to which these explanations make sense to engaged participants; and (3) the extent to which the ethnography achieves *critical* reflection on assumptions that would otherwise be taken for granted, for example, regarding how things are done, who is empowered to

Box 4.2 Features of rigorous, pragmatic ethnography (adapted from Greenhalgh and Swinglehurst 2011; Morse et al. 2002)

- Authentic immersion in the setting
- Plausible explanations
- Includes critical reflection
- Methodological coherence between the research question and methods
- Sampling sufficiency
- Iteration among sampling, data collection, and analysis
- Thinking theoretically
- Theory development

make final decisions, etc. (see Box 4.2). These criteria illuminate that rigor is integral to the entire ethnographic approach, and is not only relevant to analytic techniques. Morse and colleagues (2002) recommend five constructive procedures *during data collection* that can help to establish reliability and validity (and thereby, rigor): methodological coherence (i.e., congruence between the research question and the method(s) being used; see Chapters 2 and 3); sampling sufficiency; iterative work between sampling, data collection, and analysis; thinking theoretically; and theory development (see Box 4.2).

In Chapter 3, we share techniques and strategies for authentic immersion (criterion 1), which may be different in healthcare settings where the ethnographer(s) may be more transient. For us, immersion has the quality of "embeddedness," particularly when we are using ethnographic methods in the integrated healthcare system where we are employees. Atkins (see Foreword) and colleagues (2021) note—and we agree—that a primary aim of embedded researchers is to "demonstrate value to the health system in which they are embedded." We encourage those conducting pragmatic healthcare ethnography to practice reflexivity regarding their role(s) relative to those participating in the research: how are the researchers known to the participants and the settings, and what are ways to strengthen those ties for richer ethnography and greater value? We have all observed in our research that working in particular care settings (e.g., primary care, women's health clinics) over the course of a decade or more that our data collection has become more nuanced, and furthermore that we have established tenure and trust. Our embedded position enables our ethnographic research. Plausible explanations (criterion 2) are generated by data analysis procedures, which, as described earlier, may take any number of directions depending on the nature of the data, the parameters of the research, and the available and accessible tools. We contend that consistent work with the data, as they are being collected, helps to ensure that explanations are grounded in evidence derived from participants, even when the initial pass through the data may be more deductive and oriented toward the *a priori* research question(s). The final criterion—critical reflection—can indeed be seen as a soft dividing line between qualitative research that is or is not ethnographic, with the expectation that ethnographic work will use a critical lens to integrate and achieve holistic understanding. The case later illustrates how reflection—for example, about what is and is not apparent in the data—can lead to deeper understanding and new avenues for discovery.

Case 4

Visibility and participation in ethnographic analysis

Sarah Ono

Wouldn't it be nice to know with certainty that you are getting it right when you analyze your research data? How about finishing a project and having confidence that what you found will be put into practice clinically, or at a system level that changes a process for the better? Imagine if you could improve the odds of implementation working and proven practices getting adopted and sustained. Many of us invest our time and energy into thinking about implementation, often in systems where there are numerous barriers to change.

To illustrate the use and impact of ethnography in analysis, Sarah offers two different examples. The first highlights the unique viewpoint that an ethnographic perspective brings to thinking about data—what's there and what isn't there. The second is a case where Sarah and her team brought the study participants into the analysis process; a strategy that is more common to ethnographic research or fieldwork in an anthropology context than in a healthcare research setting. Both examples help to demonstrate ethnographic analysis as distinct from an "objective" or lab-based approach and, rather, as a process that is flexible, grounded, and likely to resonate with the study participants and others in the population of interest.

Ethnography as a methodological approach asks the researcher to center the experience of the population being studied. To pay attention to both what people say they do and what they actually do. Ethnographic analysis looks for patterns and, in doing so, takes note of outliers, considering what is explicit and also what is missing or invisible. The attention to what is not there is perhaps one of the most unique aspects of an ethnographic approach in healthcare research. In a large, multi-site VA demonstration project that tracked the implementation of the patient-centered medical home model in the VA, several of the authors in this volume contributed to the national outcomes and findings related to the implementation processes. Sarah and Dr. Samantha Solimeo were part of a research team at one of the five sites in the VA national healthcare system. They had both trained in anthropology at the same university when they were graduate students and often shared strategies when it came to research design and later analyses. The medical home model in the VA was called "PACT" or Patient-Aligned Care Teams. In the model, a patient metaphorically shares a "home" with a medical team responsible for coordination of care within the clinic and across the larger healthcare system. These were typically four-person teams in primary care that included, at minimum: a clinician, a registered nurse, a licensed practical nurse or medical support assistant, and a clerk. Sarah and Samantha collected interview and observational data for teams in various clinics covering a multi-state region in the upper Midwest. Something they both noticed independently was that the address and discussion of PACT teams tended to focus on the clinical roles: the "doctor" and the nurse. "Doctor" is here in quotes because in primary care, the clinician—frequently referred to as the "provider" in the VA health system—is often assumed to be a medical doctor (MD) and could just as likely be a physician assistant or a nurse practitioner. Regardless, people still tend to talk about the clinician as a "doctor."

For context, much of the interest in PACT implementation was focused on the model and the roles of the team central to the model that affected communication, care coordination, and delegation of responsibilities. This focus on roles was something Sarah and Samantha could anticipate and plan for in their data collection. They had data from individuals in all four of the roles making up a basic team. Sometimes teams or clinics organized themselves differently based on clinic size or coverage across multiple teams, but all roles were represented. They therefore set out to analyze their data using a conventional coding process common in qualitative health research. During the process of reviewing data and identifying initial patterns, they began to see that there was limited discussion of the clerical folks—also referred to as receptionists, schedulers, or clerks. When the role of clerks was discussed, it was different than the other roles. Not just the job of clerk and associated tasks, which were notably nonclinical in nature, but also the degree of interaction with the team was different. While everyone on a team was well aware of the clerks as key team members, it was often a role that was overlooked when talking about the team, and clerks were more often absent at meetings being observed. The clerk was also a challenging role to engage in research and data collection generally, because in the same way that they missed team meetings to staff the front desk and answer phones, they were less able to take time away from their post to participate in an interview. The role of clerks was valuable, it just wasn't understood or talked about the same way other roles were, and this absence was something Sarah and Samantha became interested in and subsequently dug into the data to understand.

To better understand the positioning and function of clerks, they needed an ethnographic approach that drew on all of the data (interview, observational, quantitative, archival, spatial), including attention to negative (or missing) data. Only when Sarah and Samantha looked holistically at what was there and what was missing could they begin to see clerks in a context that included physical spaces where work occurred, social positioning, and organizational culture. What they learned was the range of tasks that clerks performed, their frontline positioning when it came to interacting with patients, and the power they had as gatekeepers (Solimeo et al. 2017). Had they only looked at what was talked about in interviews and explicitly visible to others, they would have missed the most interesting aspects of a key role in this team-based model.

In the manuscript describing this analysis (Solimeo et al. 2017), they focused on the role of clerks on PACT teams and published it in an anthropology journal, *Medical Anthropology Quarterly*. This work was also written about for publication in *Annals of Family Medicine*, a clinical journal (Solimeo, Stewart, and Rosenthal 2016). They were able to reach two distinct audiences with the same research project and the same data. This is not possible with every study, but when it happens, it is powerful and increases the usefulness of findings by reaching different audiences. In the years since the anthropology piece was published, it has held up to readings by people in the clerk role in clinics not part of the original study. It has brought Sarah great joy to hear that upon reading the paper, even years later, people feel they "got it right" and highlighted experiences and a complexity in the work that often goes unseen and unacknowledged.

In the second example (True et al. 2021), the research team did not have to wait until the papers were published to get direct feedback from the target population in the study. In this example, Gala (see Case 3b) and Sarah used a photovoice method with veterans who experienced traumatic brain injuries (TBIs) and a family caregiver whom the veteran identified. As participatory action research, they knew from the outset that they wanted the research participants to play a role in not only the data collection but also the subsequent analysis and ongoing thinking about dissemination. In other words, they wanted the people in the study to help identify how the findings should be used to affect policy and increase awareness about the condition and the experiences of veteran families.

The study design included a series of interactions with participants individually and dyadically with their caregiver. It also provided opportunities for participants to meet each other (other veteran-caregiver dyads) to share data (photos and stories collected) and collectively contribute to the analysis of data. This was done through small group discussions, both in person and virtually. This allowed Sarah and Gala to hear from the research participants when it came to interpretations and identifying patterns in the data and provided a built-in way to check out thinking with the emic sources of data directly. The methodological approach was intended to generate trust and a richer understanding of the experience of veterans with TBIs from multiple perspectives. In situations like this, it is always interesting to see how much agreement there is among participants and also where they may disagree. These agreements and disagreements may not be completely novel to the researchers, but there is something reassuring about getting confirmation that emerging interpretations resonate with participants. Not all research designs and methodologies allow for repeat interactions and bi-directional communication with study participants, but an ethnographic approach often does, and the benefits for all involved can extend beyond the formal findings. Even in a study that is not designed to provide an intervention or deliver a treatment, benefit may be gained through the process of interacting with researchers and, in some cases, other participants, as allowable in ethnographic work. At minimum, an ethnographic approach can provide greater engagement in the process of research, and it holds the potential for supplemental learning beyond the parameters of the question at hand.

Ethnographic methods can also bring voice to individuals and populations that experience social marginalization and are minoritized. An ethnographic approach to healthcare research is more likely—if not our best bet—to be able to identify who is missing in data. If we continue to collectively only look at the data we have, missing the data that is absent, we will continue to fail entire populations not made visible in data collection and study design. The novelty of pragmatic healthcare ethnography signals the continued salience of medical anthropology and feminist theory in research on organizational culture, healthcare delivery, and the power that underlies who benefits in existing systems (Snell-Rood et al. 2021).

Part of the value in conducting research is learning new information or adding a layer of knowledge to something that we think we understand. These additions can often come from expanding research approaches to include people who are not always seen as having impact or influence on the outcomes of interest, for example, caregivers of patients in healthcare research. Unlike research conducted in a laboratory where the environment can be controlled, health services research and implementation science are strengthened when we acknowledge and allow for the introduction of complexity (Braithwaite et al. 2018). Ethnographic methods that seek to look holistically and think about what is visible and what is missing can help us to see systems and interactions with greater accuracy.

References

Atkins, David, Jeffrey T. Kullgren, and Lisa Simpson. 2021. "Enhancing the Role of Research in a Learning Health Care System." *Healthcare* 8 (June): 100556. https://doi.org/10.1016/j.hjdsi.2021.100556.

Braithwaite, Jeffrey, Kate Churruca, Janet C. Long, Louise A. Ellis, and Jessica Herkes. 2018. "When Complexity Science Meets Implementation Science: A Theoretical and Empirical Analysis of Systems Change." *BMC Medicine* 16 (1): 63. https://doi.org/10.1186/s12916-018-1057-z.

Brooks, Joanna, Serena McCluskey, Emma Turley, and Nigel King. 2015. "The Utility of Template Analysis in Qualitative Psychology Research." *Qualitative Research in Psychology* 12 (2): 202–22. https://doi.org/10.1080/14780887.2014.955224.

Brunner, Julian, Melissa M. Farmer, Bevanne Bean-Mayberry, Catherine Chanfreau-Coffinier, Claire T. Than, Alison B. Hamilton, and Erin P. Finley. 2022. "Implementing Clinical Decision Support for Reducing Women Veterans' Cardiovascular Risk in VA: A Mixed-Method, Longitudinal Study of Context, Adaptation, and Uptake." *Frontiers in Health Services* 2 (September): 946802. https://doi.org/10.3389/frhs.2022.946802.

Bunce, Arwen E., Rachel Gold, James V. Davis, Carmit K. McMullen, Victoria Jaworski, MaryBeth Mercer, and Christine Nelson. 2014. "Ethnographic Process Evaluation in Primary Care: Explaining the Complexity of Implementation." *BMC Health Services Research* 14 (1): 607. https://doi.org/10.1186/s12913-014-0607-0.

Cheney, Ann M., Christine N. Newkirk, Vhuhwavho M. Nekhavhambe, Matthew Baron Rotondi, and Alison Hamilton. 2018. "Effects of Social and Spatial Contexts on Young Latinas' Methamphetamine Use Initiation." *Journal of Ethnicity in Substance Abuse* 17 (1): 32–49. https://doi.org/10.1080/15332640.2017.1362721.

Fereday, Jennifer, and Eimear Muir-Cochrane. 2006. "Demonstrating Rigor Using Thematic Analysis: A Hybrid Approach of Inductive and Deductive Coding and Theme Development." *International Journal of Qualitative Methods* 5 (1): 80–92. https://doi.org/10.1177/160940690600500107.

Fetters, Michael D., Leslie A. Curry, and John W. Creswell. 2013. "Achieving Integration in Mixed Methods Designs-Principles and Practices." *Health Services Research* 48 (6pt2): 2134–56. https://doi.org/10.1111/1475-6773.12117.

Fix, Gemmae M., Eileen M. Dryden, Jacqueline Boudreau, Nancy R. Kressin, Allen L. Gifford, and Barbara G. Bokhour. 2021. "The Temporal Nature of Social Context: Insights from the Daily Lives of Patients with HIV." Edited by H. Jonathon Rendina. *PLOS ONE* 16 (2): e0246534. https://doi.org/10.1371/journal.pone.0246534.

Greenhalgh, Trisha, and Deborah Swinglehurst. 2011. "Studying Technology Use as Social Practice: The Untapped Potential of Ethnography." *BMC Medicine* 9 (1): 45. https://doi.org/10.1186/1741-7015-9-45.

Guetterman, Timothy C., Michael D. Fetters, and John W. Creswell. 2015. "Integrating Quantitative and Qualitative Results in Health Science Mixed Methods Research Through Joint Displays." *The Annals of Family Medicine* 13 (6): 554–61. https://doi.org/10.1370/afm.1865.

Hamilton, Alison 2012. "The Vital Conjuncture of Methamphetamine-involved Pregnancy: Objective Risks and Subjective Realities." In *Risk, Reproduction, and Narratives of Experience*, 59–77. Lauren Fordyce and Aminata Maraesa, Editors. Nashville, TN: Vanderbilt University Press.

Hamilton, Alison B., and Erin P. Finley. 2019. "Qualitative Methods in Implementation Research: An Introduction." *Psychiatry Research* 280 (October): 112516. https://doi.org/10.1016/j.psychres.2019.112516.

Hamilton, Alison, and Nicholas Goeders. 2010. "Life Trajectories of Women Methamphetamine Users with Child Sexual Abuse Histories." Presented at the Poster presentation at the 72nd annual scientific meeting of the College on Problems of Drug Dependence, Scottsdale, AZ, June.

Ilott, Irene, Kate Gerrish, Sabrina A. Eltringham, Carolyn Taylor, and Sue Pownall. 2016. "Exploring Factors That Influence the Spread and Sustainability of a Dysphagia Innovation: An Instrumental Case Study." *BMC Health Services Research* 16 (1): 406. https://doi.org/10.1186/s12913-016-1653-6.

Johnson-Hanks, Jennifer. 2002. "On the Limits of Life Stages in Ethnography: Toward a Theory of Vital Conjunctures." *American Anthropologist* 104 (3): 865–80. https://doi.org/10.1525/aa.2002.104.3.865.

King, Nigel 2012. "Doing Template Analysis." In *Qualitative Organizational Research*, edited by Gillian Symon and Catherine Cassell, 426–50. London: Sage.

Lee, Kellyn, and Ruth Bartlett. 2021. "Material Citizenship: An Ethnographic Study Exploring Object–Person Relations in the Context of People with Dementia in Care Homes." *Sociology of Health and Illness* 43 (6): 1471–85. https://doi.org/10.1111/1467-9566.13321.

Lewinski, Allison A., Matthew J. Crowley, Christopher Miller, Hayden B. Bosworth, George L. Jackson, Karen Steinhauser, Courtney White-Clark, Felicia McCant, and Leah L. Zullig. 2021. "Applied Rapid Qualitative Analysis to Develop a Contextually Appropriate Intervention and Increase the Likelihood of Uptake." *Medical Care* 59 (Suppl 3): S242–51. https://doi.org/10.1097/MLR.0000000000001553.

Maietta, Raymond, Paul Mihas, Kevin Swartout, Jeff Petruzzelli, and Alison Hamilton. 2021. "Sort and Sift, Think and Shift: Let the Data Be Your Guide an Applied Approach to Working With, Learning From, and Privileging Qualitative Data." *The Qualitative Report* 26 (6): 2045–60. https://doi.org/10.46743/2160-3715/2021.5013.

Maietta, Raymond, E. J. Reifstek, Jeff Petruzzelli, Paul Mihas, Kevin Swartout, and Alison Hamilton. 2024. "The Sort and Sift, Think and Shift Analysis Method." In *Qualitative Research and Evaluation in Physical Education and Sport Pedagogy*, edited by Kevin Andrew Richards, Michael A. Hemphill, and Paul M. Wright. Burlington, MA: Jones & Bartlett Learning.

Meyer, Daniel Z., and Leanne M. Avery. 2009. "Excel as a Qualitative Data Analysis Tool." *Field Methods* 21 (1): 91–112. https://doi.org/10.1177/1525822X08323985.

Miller, William L., Benjamin F. Crabtree, Michael I. Harrison, and Mary L. Fennell. 2013. "Integrating Mixed Methods in Health Services and Delivery System Research." *Health Services Research* 48 (6pt2): 2125–33. https://doi.org/10.1111/1475-6773.12123.

Morse, Janice M., ed. 2017. *Analyzing and Conceptualizing the Theoretical Foundations of Nursing*. New York: Springer Publishing Company.

Morse, Janice M., Michael Barrett, Maria Mayan, Karin Olson, and Jude Spiers. 2002. "Verification Strategies for Establishing Reliability and Validity in Qualitative Research." *International Journal of Qualitative Methods* 1 (2): 13–22.

Nevedal, Andrea L., Caitlin M. Reardon, Marilla A. Opra Widerquist, George L. Jackson, Sarah L. Cutrona, Brandolyn S. White, and Laura J. Damschroder. 2021. "Rapid versus Traditional Qualitative Analysis Using the Consolidated Framework for Implementation Research (CFIR)." *Implementation Science* 16 (1): 67. https://doi.org/10.1186/s13012-021-01111-5.

Obert, Jeanne L., Alison Hamilton Brown, Joan Zweben, Darrell Christian, Jenn Delmhorst, Sam Minsky, Patrick Morrisey, Denna Vandersloot, and Ahndrea Weiner. 2005. "When Treatment Meets Research: Clinical Perspectives from the CSAT Methamphetamine Treatment Project." *Journal of Substance Abuse Treatment* 28 (3): 231–37. https://doi.org/10.1016/j.jsat.2004.12.008.

Palinkas, Lawrence A. 2014. "Qualitative and Mixed Methods in Mental Health Services and Implementation Research." *Journal of Clinical Child & Adolescent Psychology* 43 (6): 851–61. https://doi.org/10.1080/15374416.2014.910791.

Palinkas, Lawrence A., Sapna J. Mendon, and Alison B. Hamilton. 2019. "Innovations in Mixed Methods Evaluations." *Annual Review of Public Health* 40 (1): 423–42. https://doi.org/10.1146/annurev-publhealth-040218-044215.

Palinkas, Lawrence A., and Douglas Zatzick. 2019. "Rapid Assessment Procedure Informed Clinical Ethnography (RAPICE) in Pragmatic Clinical Trials of Mental Health Services Implementation: Methods and Applied Case Study." *Administration and Policy in Mental Health and Mental Health Services Research* 46 (2): 255–70. https://doi.org/10.1007/s10488-018-0909-3.

Proudfoot, Kevin. 2023. "Inductive/Deductive Hybrid Thematic Analysis in Mixed Methods Research." *Journal of Mixed Methods Research* 17 (3): 308–26. https://doi.org/10.1177/15586898221126816.

Ritchie, Jane, and Liz Spencer. 1994. "Qualitative Data Analysis for Applied Policy Research." In *Analyzing Qualitative Data*, edited by Alan Bryman and Robert G. Burgess, 173–94. Abingdon, UK: Taylor & Francis. https://doi.org/10.4324/9780203413081_chapter_9.

Ryan, Gery W., and H. Russell Bernard. 2003. "Techniques to Identify Themes." *Field Methods* 15 (1): 85–109. https://doi.org/10.1177/1525822X02239569.

Snell-Rood, Claire, Elise Trott Jaramillo, Alison B. Hamilton, Sarah E. Raskin, Francesca M. Nicosia, and Cathleen Willging. 2021. "Advancing Health Equity through a Theoretically Critical Implementation Science." *Translational Behavioral Medicine* 11 (8): 1617–25. https://doi.org/10.1093/tbm/ibab008.

Solimeo, Samantha L., Sarah S. Ono, Kenda R. Stewart, Michelle A. Lampman, Gary E. Rosenthal, and Greg L. Stewart. 2017. "Gatekeepers as Care Providers: The Care Work of Patient-centered Medical Home Clerical Staff." *Medical Anthropology Quarterly* 31 (1): 97–114. https://doi.org/10.1111/maq.12281.

Solimeo, Samantha L., Greg L. Stewart, and Gary E. Rosenthal. 2016. "The Critical Role of Clerks in the Patient-Centered Medical Home." *The Annals of Family Medicine* 14 (4): 377–79. https://doi.org/10.1370/afm.1934.

St. George, Sara M., Audrey R. Harkness, Carlos E. Rodriguez-Diaz, Elliott R. Weinstein, Vanina Pavia, and Alison B. Hamilton. 2023. "Applying Rapid Qualitative Analysis for Health Equity: Lessons Learned Using 'EARS' With Latino Communities." *International Journal of Qualitative Methods* 22 (January): 160940692311649. https://doi.org/10.1177/16094069231164938.

Taylor, Beck, Catherine Henshall, Sara Kenyon, Ian Litchfield, and Sheila Greenfield. 2018. "Can Rapid Approaches to Qualitative Analysis Deliver Timely, Valid Findings to Clinical Leaders? A Mixed Methods Study Comparing Rapid and Thematic Analysis." *BMJ Open* 8 (10): e019993. https://doi.org/10.1136/bmjopen-2017-019993.

True, Gala, Lawrence Davidson, Ray Facundo, David V. Meyer, Sharon Urbina, and Sarah S. Ono. 2021. "'Institutions Don't Hug People': A Roadmap for Building Trust, Connectedness, and Purpose through Photovoice Collaboration." *Journal of Humanistic Psychology* 61 (3): 365–404. https://doi.org/10.1177/0022167819853344.

Urquhart, Lynn M., Jean S. Ker, and Charlotte E. Rees. 2018. "Exploring the Influence of Context on Feedback at Medical School: A Video-Ethnography Study." *Advances in Health Sciences Education* 23 (1): 159–86. https://doi.org/10.1007/s10459-017-9781-2.

Van Belle, Elise, Jeltje Giesen, Tiffany Conroy, Marloes Van Mierlo, Hester Vermeulen, Getty Huisman-de Waal, and Maud Heinen. 2020. "Exploring Person-centred Fundamental Nursing Care in Hospital Wards: A Multi-site Ethnography." *Journal of Clinical Nursing* 29 (11–12): 1933–44. https://doi.org/10.1111/jocn.15024.

CHAPTER 5

Sharing ethnographic findings

Introduction

Writing is inherent to the definition of ethnography ("to write people"). Part of the ethnographic process from the beginning, writing is how we document, analyze, and disseminate what we have learned in relation to—and likely beyond—the research question(s) (Montagnes, Montagnes, and Yang 2022; Schindler and Schäfer 2021). Writing often starts with fieldnotes, recording what is observed and reflecting on our observations in memos (see Chapter 3). Writing facilitates analysis and helps to formulate and synthesize ideas into a cogent argument. Just as we think about analysis early and often (see Chapter 4), we think about writing up insights early and often, including early and consistent considerations of audience, format, and dissemination goals. In pragmatic healthcare ethnography, dissemination is likely to extend beyond academic products, where accessibility and impacts may be limited. Thinking about what you want to share, the key data sources and the insights they provide, as well as who the key audiences are, can help a research team navigate the writing process (see Figure 5.1). In this chapter, we discuss practical strategies for developing products from ethnographic work, with the goal of making findings available and accessible to a variety of audiences in a variety of formats.

Getting started: What do we want to share?

In Chapter 4, we describe using a variety of analytic tools to develop a holistic understanding of what we are studying in our ethnography. With a foundation of deep familiarization with our data, tools like memoing, diagramming, and coding move us toward synthesis and readiness to share what we have learned, potentially with a variety of audiences. Given that we typically have multiple sources of data in our ethnography, one of the first challenges we may face is deciding what to focus on in a given product. In pragmatic work, *we prioritize sharing information that can inform a change in practice, policy, or mindset*. In some cases, this decision may be based on what we have been asked to do by a particular constituent.

DOI: 10.4324/9781003390657-5

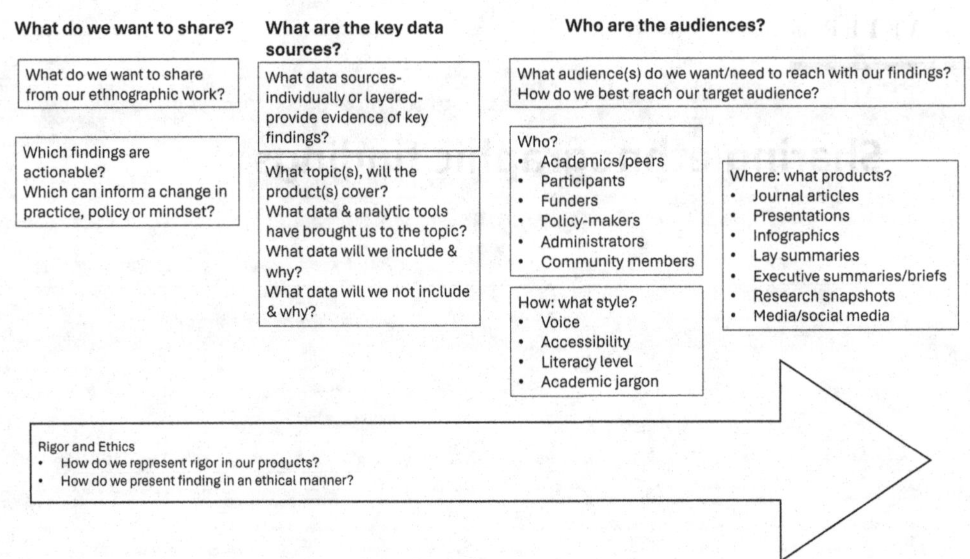

Figure 5.1 Thinking through sharing ethnographic findings

In the VA, we are often asked by national-level partners, who are responsible for establishing and monitoring practice and policy, to study things that are happening (or not happening) in the healthcare system. For example, Alison and her team were asked by national women's health partners to study harassment of women veterans, after a survey had found that one in four women was experiencing harassment while on VA grounds (Klap et al. 2019). Because of the complexity of the problem, Alison and her team used multiple methods for a set of related projects, including individual interviews, focus groups, public deliberation groups, observations, expert panels, and surveys. Findings from all of these methods could not be included in a single product, and the implications of the work were different for different audiences. The team prioritized identifying and delivering key messages from the findings in straightforward presentations and reports for the partners, as they were the primary constituent responsible for addressing this problem within the healthcare system in a timely and effective manner. This meant sharing with the partners what was learned about veterans' and staff experiences with and perceptions of harassment (what was the nature of the experiences, who was perpetrating harassment, where was it happening), what actions (if any) were taken in response to harassment, and what recommendations were given for eliminating and preventing harassment. The process of analyzing data for this purpose was relatively straightforward. The team had purposefully designed several of their data collection approaches to elicit this information, with the advanced knowledge that it would be needed, and needed quickly and reliably. Findings that they reported to the partners informed the development of anti-harassment policies and campaigns that continue to this day. In addition, findings synthesized across multiple data sources were disseminated via journal articles (Dyer et al. 2019; Fenwick et al. 2021; Fenwick et al. 2021), conference presentations, lay summaries, research snapshots, and social media. To sum up, Alison and her team got started with sharing their findings by focusing on what data and findings they had available, what their priority audience needed, what format(s) would align with that audience's needs, what data and key messages would meet those needs, and what impacts they were intending to have. This approach to sharing findings illustrates the pragmatism that we emphasize throughout this book, as we define in Chapter 1: "keeping our focus on issues and data relevant for making decisions and taking action" (Glasgow 2013).

Building on our data sources and analytic resources

As we describe in Chapter 4, many of the resources that we develop and use to understand our data throughout analysis—memos, tables, diagrams, maps—often become vehicles for communicating our findings. Usually, we first ground this process in a clear understanding of what types of data are available and will be used for a given product. Ethnographic writing typically combines, or "layers," several sources of data such as interviews, observations, and archival documents, potentially alongside other types of data such as surveys or administrative data. As we describe and illustrate in Chapter 2, it is helpful to have the data sources laid out in a table and to reference that table when we're starting to write; this reinforces the value of "getting organized" in the early stages of analysis (Chapter 4). Furthermore, data summary tables are helpful in final products to orient the audience to the nature of the data and findings being presented. Writing can be shared across the team. We often have one person on the writing team work on refining and finalizing data summary tables for the methods section of a journal article while other members of the team work on other sections.

In preparing to write (or otherwise share findings), we also want to make sure to capitalize on all of the hard work that has been accomplished, "mining" our analytic resources to make decisions about what findings we plan to share and what key messages we want to impart. In Gemmae's ethnographic study of HIV care (Fix et al. 2018), she and her colleagues wanted to write about the relationship between how clinicians thought about their patients and the specific practice setting of the HIV clinic. During analysis, Gemmae systematically reviewed fieldnotes for each of the eight HIV clinics, looking for information about how clinicians talked about their patients, and began to notice patterns. She also looked for divergent cases where the data might contradict her theory on the relationship between clinicians' conceptualizations of patients and site context. An early version of Table 5.1 was an analytic tool to begin exploring the patterns between team composition and how HIV clinicians talked about and conceptualized their patients.

In the writing process, the interview and observation data were brought together to demonstrate how the ways in which clinicians viewed their patients were related to the clinics' culture and how the clinics' culture reflected both who was on the HIV care team and the interactions among team members. This insight was shared, first at an academic conference and later in a journal article detailing variation in HIV care team setting and culture (Fix et al. 2018). The tables used initially for analysis were incorporated into the publication, which reinforced the transparency and rigor of the analytic process. And because the interviews and fieldnotes were the origin of the insight, fieldnotes were included on an introductory slide at the academic conference and in the methods of the resulting paper as an entree into the findings, which included snippets from observation fieldnotes and interviews. Excerpts of fieldnotes and observations can and should be included in the resulting product(s), just like interview or focus group data are often included in qualitative products. It is this data that provides authentic, holistic, and grounded insight into the lived experiences of the study's participants.

Table 5.1 Team composition and clinician conceptualization of patient behavior (Fix et al. 2018)

Site	*Team composition*						*Degree of interaction across professionals*	*Clinician conceptualization of the basis for patient self-management*
	*Clinicians (MD, NP, PA)**	*Nurses*	*LPN* and med. support asst.*	*Pharmacist*	*Mental Health*	*Social Work*		
1	3	1	—	—	—	—	Low	Individual Responsibility
3	4*	1	—	1	—	—	Low	Individual Responsibility
4	6*	1	—	2	—	—	Moderate	Individual Responsibility
6	4*	2	1	1	—	—	Moderate	Individual Responsibility
5	2	—	—	1	1	—	Moderate (w/dyads)	Pt/clinician dependent
2	4*	1	—	1	1	—	High	Socio-culturally embedded
7	4*	1	—	1	1	1**	High	Socio-culturally embedded
8	6	1	3	2	—	1	High	Socio-culturally embedded

Nurse Practitioner (NP); Physician's Assistant (PA); Licensed Professional Nurse (LPN). *Site has a training program. **Plus 2 case managers.

Ethnographic writing is traditionally descriptive, with rich details, strong evidence for claims, and humanizing stories that can be powerful, illustrative, and resonant with readers. In Erin's ethnography of post-traumatic stress disorder (PTSD) among veterans of the wars in Iraq and Afghanistan, she included a chapter on veterans' war stories early in the book as a way of bringing readers into the events that led to a PTSD diagnosis and veterans' efforts to navigate healthcare in the aftermath. Stories are a deep and immediate way of conveying information and can inspire readers to think in entirely new ways. Although not all ethnographic studies will be written in a format that includes stories, ethnographic analysis and writing can invite consideration of novel ways to present data—as in the use of veteran profiles in Meg's Chapter 2 case study or even the use of ethnographic "poems" crafted from compiling participants' written text messages (Creese et al. 2023).

Reaching our target audience(s)

Selecting journals and publishing ethnographic work

Publications in health-related journals are perhaps the main way that researchers share findings from our ethnographic studies. As with qualitative research more broadly, ethnographic research tends not to be published in "top-tier" journals with high impact factors, reflecting a widespread bias toward quantitative research. In 2016, in response to

The BMJ's rejection of qualitative research on the grounds of low priority, Dr. Trisha Greenhalgh and 75 other academics from 11 countries wrote an open letter urging the journal to revise their policy, pointing out several impactful qualitative papers published by the journal (Greenhalgh et al. 2016). This letter prompted several responses, including a paper in the *International Journal of Qualitative Methods*, "Five tips for writing qualitative research in high-impact journals: moving from #BMJnoQual" (Clark and Thompson 2016). Their tips, which resonate greatly with us, are as follows: (1) try, try, try again (to get your work accepted in high-quality journals with your target audience); (2) nail your key messages; (3) match your messages to the audience of your targeted journals; (4) tune into the journal and its aims and scope; and (5) remember you are doing community work. These tips remain relevant beyond academic publishing. As we note earlier, Alison and her team working on the harassment-related research had to continually hone in on actionable messages from their findings for their primary audience for the work to be useful and impactful.

In addition to the challenge of publishing qualitative papers in prominent journals, ethnographers hoping to write for academic audiences have the challenge of publishing multimethod research. Almost two decades ago, Stange (2006) noted limitations to the dissemination of results from mixed methods studies, with studies publishing different results from different methods, in different journals. Their solutions to this problem remain relevant today: (1) publish quantitative and qualitative papers in separate journals, but with references and links to the companion papers; (2) publish concurrent or sequential quantitative and qualitative papers in the same journal; (3) publish an integrated article, possibly with appendices that describe method details; (4) co-publish separate quantitative and qualitative papers with another paper that draws lessons from the analyses; and (5) develop an online discussion of readers and commentators to foster cross-disciplinary communities of knowledge.

As Sarah describes in her Chapter 4 case study, our colleague, Dr. Samantha Solimeo, used yet another approach. Samantha wrote about the same ethnographic project for two very different academic audiences: social science and clinical. In one paper, written for a social science audience via *Medical Anthropology Quarterly*, she described the important role of clerks in patient-centered medical homes (Solimeo et al. 2017). As is typical in this genre, she began with an excerpt from an interview with a nurse describing all of the work clerks do. In speaking about this paper with a clinical colleague, Samatha realized she could share this same insight with a clinical audience (Solimeo, Stewart, and Rosenthal 2016). She wrote a "Discussion" piece for a clinical audience via *The Annals of Family Medicine* about this same phenomenon, but in a more structured, less narrative format.

With these tips and suggestions in mind, we can consider a wide range of publishing options, re-emphasizing the importance of thinking about the combination of our key messages (derived from our findings) and our audience of interest. We and our colleagues have published health-related ethnographic work in a wide range of journals, including but not limited to the journals in Box 5.1.

There are several strategies to identify a journal. We recommend asking colleagues for journal recommendations, identifying where papers similar to the manuscript in preparation are published, as well as reviewing your own references to see what literature you are situating your work. Additionally, tools like the "Journal Author Name Estimator" (JANE) website can identify potential journals, or searching for where similar

Box 5.1 Journals that publish ethnographic findings

- *Administration and Policy in Mental Health and Mental Health Services Research*
- *Annals of Family Medicine*
- *BMC Health Services Research*
- *BMJ Global Health*
- *BMJ Open*
- *Global Public Health*
- *Human Organization*
- *Implementation Science*
- *JAMA Internal Medicine*
- *Journal of Community Health*
- *Journal of Community Psychology*
- *Journal of Contemporary Ethnography*
- *Journal of General Internal Medicine*
- *Journal of Healthcare for the Poor and Underserved*
- *Journal of Humanistic Psychology*
- *Medical Anthropology Quarterly*
- *Medical Care*
- *Patient Education and Counseling*
- *PEC Innovation*
- *PLoS Global Public Health*
- *PLoS One*
- *Psychiatric Services*
- *Qualitative Health Research*
- *Qualitative Research*
- *Social Science and Medicine*
- *Sociology of Health & Illness*

topics have been published in an academic database such as PubMed or Google Scholar can offer a window into journals that might be a good fit.

When considering a journal, it is particularly important to examine the journal's norms for presenting results. Most medical journals adhere to a relatively formal structure, with only findings in the results sections. In contrast, social science journals may encourage the integration of results and interpretation/discussion throughout. It is important to consider each journal's norms for describing methods and results, and any content specifications, such as expectations for theoretical grounding. For example, *Social Science and Medicine* states the following about theoretical engagement: "We expect the authors to provide a self-sustained argument, accessible to nonexperts, that situates the manuscript within a relevant literature and offers a distinct added value. A telltale sign of weak theoretical engagement is theoretical obfuscation or the mere illustration or application of existing concepts" (Timmermans 2012). Journals often have submission guidelines for prospective authors on their website. These specify their aim and scope, word count, and other factors that can inform whether that particular journal is a good fit.

Anthropologists have a long and robust history of publishing their ethnographies in the form of books and book chapters. These formats are another option for publishing ethnographic findings. Books and book chapters are appealing because they provide more space to explore and expound on findings, although from a pragmatic perspective, it is unlikely that we will have time, funding, or energy to write books in the context of busy studies. Additionally, it is unlikely that our clinical, policy, or academic medicine audiences will readily access books and use them (as they might use journal articles) to inform change efforts. However, ethnographic books written in a more popular format, such as Arthur Kleinman's classic *The Illness Narratives*, Svea Closser's *Chasing Polio in Pakistan*, or Erin's *Fields of Combat*, can make in-depth findings on important challenges accessible to a wider audience.

Presenting ethnographic work to academic audiences

Conference presentations, both oral and poster formats, can be a helpful strategy to move an early idea into a product. Conference abstracts are typically between 200 and 750 words. This short format can be an easy way to begin articulating an idea. We often push ourselves and our team members to submit evolving ideas as abstracts for conferences. This can help solidify ideas and build momentum toward writing articles. Abstracts follow similar formats to manuscripts, but in a much briefer form. Accepted abstracts are invited for presentation, typically in poster or oral formats. Poster presentations offer a large, one-view opportunity to describe a study. They typically have five or six sections: Background, Objective, Methods, Results, Conclusions, and sometimes Implications for Practice.

For example, Gemmae and her team decided to organize their findings about HIV clinic variations into the seven features of a patient-centered medical home: patient-driven, team-based, efficient, comprehensive, continuous, coordinated, and good communication (Jackson et al. 2013). For the poster, a table was used to show the audience how HIV clinics varied in terms of these features. Visuals are powerful communicators of ethnographic findings in posters, which attendees often only glance at while moving through poster sessions. Oral presentations follow a format similar to posters but are often presented through a series of slides, usually within 10–15-minute time blocks. Academic conferences are full of potential consumers of later papers. They also present an opportunity to get feedback on the product and key messages, which can be refined for later products such as journal articles or reports.

Preparing nonacademic products

Different audiences will gravitate toward, prioritize, and resonate with different types of products, as illustrated in Table 5.2. Of course, audiences can and do engage with varied products, but accessibility can be challenging if there are paywalls preventing access to journal articles or if work is written in an inaccessible voice, full of jargon, or at an inappropriate literacy level. In writing up our pragmatic healthcare ethnographic work, we find that we are constantly having to expand our notions of audience, particularly when thinking about writing for audiences who may not be familiar with or see the value in ethnography. Increasingly we are called upon to get creative (and proficient) with formats beyond traditional academic products, as we explore further later in this chapter.

Table 5.2 Audiences and common products for ethnographic findings

Audience	*Common products*
Academic researchers	Journal articles Book chapters and books Oral and poster presentations at conferences
Leadership, operations, or clinical partners	Executive summary or brief White paper Brief "high-level" presentation
Funders	Executive summaries, briefs, white papers, and/or technical reports
Study participants, community members, or general public	Lay summary Infographics Social media, video, and podcast

Leaders, clinical and operations partners, and funders may prefer, and even require, *executive summaries*, *briefs*, *white papers*, and/or *technical reports*. In our experience, these types of products rarely contain extensive information about the methods used to generate the findings, though this information may be placed in an appendix or supplement (and should at least be available in a concise and accurate form, if requested). They also do not tend to be replete with findings, instead focusing on "big picture" takeaways from the work, and perhaps select quotations that illustrate key points in an evocative manner. We have been frequently invited to do brief *presentations* and *lay summaries* for these and other constituents (e.g., patients, clinicians) who may be less likely to read academic journal articles. As with reports and briefs, accessibility is key, with an emphasis on the implications of the ethnographic findings, tailored to the particular audience. Alison frequently shares findings of ethnographic projects with operations partners, presenting both findings pertaining to the partners' priorities (like the harassment example described earlier) and unexpected or "surprising" findings that may become directions for future projects. We have also been asked to prepare presentations for our partners to share independently of the research team. Creating a product for someone else's use again requires careful consideration of how results are presented in a rigorous and ethical manner, which we explore further later in this chapter.

Infographics and other types of *visual displays* are increasingly popular, sometimes even being requested by journals for dissemination via social media. Visual summaries of findings provide an accessible, engaging format that can be shared with a wide variety of audiences.

On a project about the implementation of a new electronic health record (EHR), Gemmae wanted to learn how the healthcare system could prepare patients for the new EHR, including what patients should know. She designed a two-part study to learn patients' perspectives and experiences. In the first phase, Gemmae conducted a "listening tour." She met with four patient advisory groups from across the United States. The goal of these discussions was to explore the needs of patients in anticipation of the EHR transition. After the tour was complete, Gemmae's team created a one-page summary to share back with the patient advisory groups (see Figure 5.2). The summary was specifically designed with the patient advisory groups in mind. Instead of an academic "Background," there was a paragraph on "What is happening?" The "Methods" instead asked "What did we do?" and "What did we ask?" The summary was easy to read and

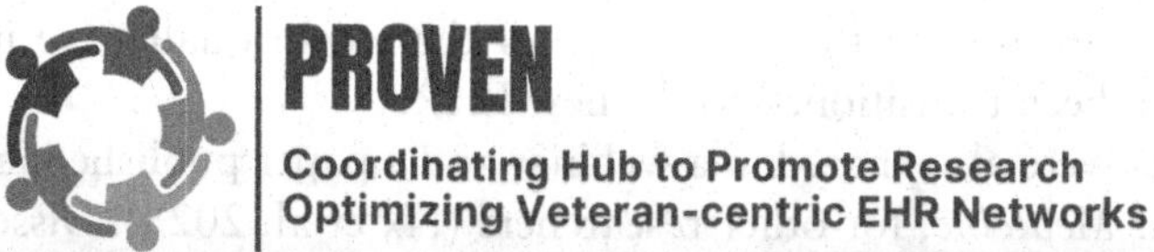

Supporting Veterans through Electronic Health Record Transitions

A LISTENING TOUR OF VETERAN ENGAGEMENT GROUPS

WHAT IS HAPPENING?

The Department of Veterans Affairs (VA) has embarked on the largest system-wide electronic health record (EHR) transition in history. Our goal is to understand Veterans' transition-related needs and priorities, and to identify strategies to support Veterans prior to and during the transition.

WHAT DID WE DO?

Listening Sessions

We conducted listening sessions with four Veteran Engagement Groups around the country between January and March 2022. The groups ranged from 3 to 13 members and discussions lasted 60 to 90 minutes.

WHAT DID WE ASK?

We asked...

- What have you heard or read about the transition to the new EHR?
- What do Veterans need to know about the transition?
- How can the VA help Veterans during the transition?

WHAT DID WE FIND?

"When this transition happens, I need someone who will walk me through it when I'm having a rough time."

Guidance on patient portals across users and roles

Veterans suggested the need for...

- "Dummy" accounts to practice using the new software
- Peer navigators to help answer questions and educate
- Tools to refer patients to resources (e.g., help line or online chat)
- Ensuring community organizations have the resources and information about the transition to share (especially in rural areas)

Avoid "over promising and under-performing" by "putting the bottom line up front" to instill confidence in the VA.

Building and maintaining trust

It is important to provide clear, direct VA communications to build and maintain trust. Veterans need to know...

- Why the system is changing
- When changes will happen
- What to expect
- How the VA will protect patient data

Keep communications "short and simple" and provide "happy, healthy" messages about the transition.

Advertising and marketing strategies

Veterans suggested ways to spread news about the transition like...

- Digital messages (e.g., email or through My HealtheVet)
- Print (e.g., flyers)
- Word-of-mouth (e.g., via providers)
- Television or radio advertisements
- Providing information packets to community partners

Funded by VA HSR&D. Study number SDR 197-20-8

March 2022 www.hsrd.research.va.gov/centers/proven | 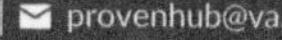 provenhub@va.gov | 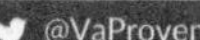 @VaProven

Figure 5.2 Summary for patient advisory groups

included the three main takeaways. These same takeaways were then used to develop the interview guides used in the next phase of the work: qualitative interviews with patients who had been transitioned to the new EHR.

Study findings were also shared in a webinar and a paper published in the *Journal of General Internal Medicine*, for other researchers (Fix et al. 2023). Disseminating findings to an array of audiences using these different channels enabled the work to reach a much wider audience. Research teams can even consider structured approaches like community-engaged research dissemination planning (Cunningham-Erves et al. 2020) to identify which findings are most critical to share, with whom, and in what formats.

Social media, *videos*, and *podcasts* can help spread findings to a much broader, even global audience. The specific social media will likely continue to change, but the principle of simplifying to key points is the same across formats. Podcasts provide a similarly accessible format by giving a verbal summary of key insights. Podcasts can easily be shared on websites or social media. Alison, Gemmae, and Erin have each collaboratively and independently shared their work through webinars with others interested in using pragmatic ethnographic methods in their health research. The most notable of these was a webinar on "Qualitative Methods in Rapid Turn-Around Health Services Research" (Hamilton 2013), which has been cited in over 300 publications across a wide variety of disciplines.

Demonstrating rigor

A chapter about sharing ethnographic findings would not be complete without considering rigor and ethics. Audiences want to be able to trust the information they hear or read. Rigor can be demonstrated in ethnographic work through clear descriptions of the process and methods the research team used. In ethnographic writing, as in analysis (see Chapter 4), it is important to "stay close to the data." This means that the presentation of findings should accurately represent what people shared in interviews or focus groups, and/or what was ethnographically observed. One strategy to keep the writing reflective of the data is to pull in key excerpts to anchor the writing to specific examples. In pragmatic ethnographic writing, we often select our writing tasks by revisiting the research question and the audience in order to consider what data will be most relevant to present and the format for that presentation. We can use our research question memos and/or our topic memos to think through the scope, potentially using outlines or other visuals (e.g., diagrams) to map out the writing plan. These approaches enhance rigor by building on available, accumulated evidence and being transparent about how we move from data to product. Transparency contributes to trustworthiness, a hallmark of rigorous qualitative research (Lincoln and Guba 1985).

Earlier in this chapter we described how Gemmae and her team organize their poster presentation of findings from her ethnographic study of HIV care, using the seven features of a patient-centered medical home. Gemmae used the seven features to structure the analysis and then the resulting paper. Each feature of a patient-centered medical home (e.g., patient-driven) was accompanied by exemplary quotes. As Gemmae wrote the manuscript, she kept these quotes in a comment so she could reference them and stay close to the data as she wrote (see Figure 5.3). This final paper was published in a special issue of the *Journal of General Internal Medicine*.

This example demonstrates the value of having a rubric (the seven features) by which to explore and organize findings, when a relevant rubric is available and appropriate.

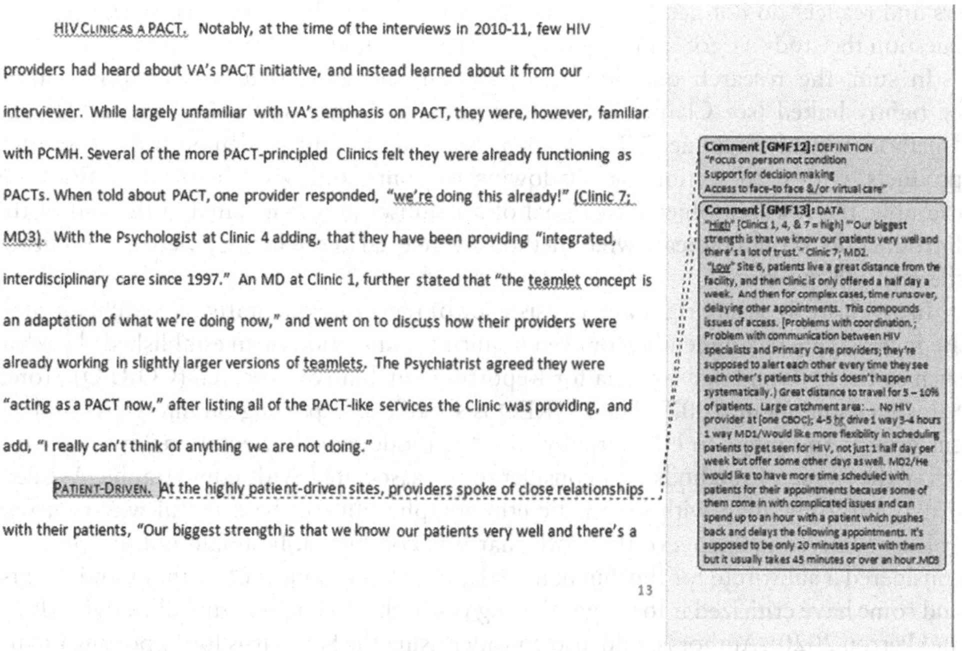

HIV CLINIC AS A PACT. Notably, at the time of the interviews in 2010-11, few HIV providers had heard about VA's PACT initiative, and instead learned about it from our interviewer. While largely unfamiliar with VA's emphasis on PACT, they were, however, familiar with PCMH. Several of the more PACT-principled Clinics felt they were already functioning as PACTs. When told about PACT, one provider responded, "we're doing this already!" (Clinic 7; MD3). With the Psychologist at Clinic 4 adding, that they have been providing "integrated, interdisciplinary care since 1997." An MD at Clinic 1, further stated that "the teamlet concept is an adaptation of what we're doing now," and went on to discuss how their providers were already working in slightly larger versions of teamlets. The Psychiatrist agreed they were "acting as a PACT now," after listing all of the PACT-like services the Clinic was providing, and add, "I really can't think of anything we are not doing."

PATIENT-DRIVEN. At the highly patient-driven sites, providers spoke of close relationships with their patients, "Our biggest strength is that we know our patients very well and there's a

13

Comment [GMF12]: DEFINITION
"Focus on person not condition
Support for decision making
Access to face-to face &/or virtual care"

Comment [GMF13]: DATA
"High" [Clinics 1, 4, & 7 = high] "Our biggest strength is that we know our patients very well and there's a lot of trust." Clinic 7; MD2.
"Low" Site 6, patients live a great distance from the facility, and then Clinic is only offered a half day a week. And then for complex cases, time runs over, delaying other appointments. This compounds issues of access. [Problems with coordination.; Problem with communication between HIV specialists and Primary Care providers; they're supposed to alert each other every time they see each other's patients but this doesn't happen systematically.) Great distance to travel for 5 – 10% of patients. Large catchment area: ... No HIV provider at [one CBOC]; 4-5 hr drive 1 way 3-4 hours 1 way MD1/Would like more flexibility in scheduling patients to get seen for HIV, not just 1 half day per week but offer some other days as well. MD2/He would like to have more time scheduled with patients for their appointments because some of them come in with complicated issues and can spend up to an hour with a patient which pushes back and delays the following appointments. It's supposed to be only 20 minutes spent with them but it usually takes 45 minutes or over an hour.MD3

Figure 5.3 Paper draft in progress using data to support the narrative

Similarly, when Alison was thinking about writing up what she was learning about attitudes toward manualized treatment for methamphetamine dependence (see Chapter 4), she found a helpful theory-based rubric about practitioners' concerns about these treatments, divided into six broad categories: (1) the therapeutic relationship; (2) patient/client needs; (3) competence and job satisfaction; (4) credibility; (5) restriction of clinical innovation; and (6) feasibility issues (Addis, Wade, and Hatgis 1999). These categories were a good "fit" for the data Alison had collected and worked well as a way to organize and present the findings (Obert et al. 2005). Not all ethnographic writing will feature theory, but engagement with theory during the course of ethnographic work is considered to be another hallmark of rigor (Morse et al. 2002).

Another core component of rigor in writing up ethnographic work is the description of the methods. This is the what, how, and when information was collected, from whom and where, and the process by which the team arrived at the interpretation. Different products have different norms for how much detail is needed about methods. In a journal article, information about the research process goes in the methods section and is described using discipline-specific terminology. This section should be specific to how the ethnography was conducted. If only some of the ethnographic data are being drawn on in a particular product, that decision needs to be explained. Furthermore, methods that are reported on should be consistent with the findings that are presented. For example, if the team reports that they used observational methods and took fieldnotes to document their observations, the results should include findings from the fieldnotes. As a rule of thumb, if the methods are so generic that they can be copied and pasted into a product from a different study and still be accurate, there is not enough specificity. A statement such as "we conducted and analyzed qualitative interviews" is never sufficient. If reviewers and readers do not get a clear enough sense of how the work was done, they may question the study's rigor and they may not trust the findings.

In sum, the research question, study design, methods used, and analysis should be tightly linked (see Chapter 2)—achieving what Morse and colleagues (2002) call "methodological coherence." These linkages are important to demonstrate in written products, with each section foreshadowing or connecting with the next section. For example, the research objective or goal of a manuscript, often stated at the end of the Introduction, should indicate what methods were used and why they were a good fit for the research question.

In an effort to ensure rigor and consistency of reporting qualitative research, journals are increasingly recommending or even requiring completion of an established checklist, such as the Consolidated Criteria for Reporting Qualitative Research (COREQ) (Tong, Sainsbury, and Craig 2007). The COREQ is specific to reporting on interviews and focus groups and refers to ethnography as a "methodological orientation," but does not cover the range of methods and considerations associated with ethnography. As such, it may not fully align with pragmatic ethnography but can be a useful way to assess at least some components of the work that was conducted. It should not, however, be considered a substitute for thorough, holistic, rigorous accounts of methods and results, and some have criticized it for depoliticizing research and emphasizing objectivity (Buus and Perron 2020). Authors could also consider using the Standards for Reporting Qualitative Research (SRQR), which offers a more open-ended way of describing how the study was conducted (O'Brien et al. 2014). In our experience, if this or another checklist is required, we as authors have often indicated what aspects of the checklist are not applicable, with an accompanying rationale if requested. Additionally, though dated in some ways, Michael Quinn Patton's 2003 Qualitative Evaluation Checklist contains extensive guidance on qualitative methods, including ethnographic fieldwork, and may be a useful tool for ethnographers to explore (Patton 2003). To the best of our knowledge, there is not a checklist specific to ethnography, though there are guidelines for conducting meta-ethnography (Cahill et al. 2018). Any rubric should be considered a helpful tool to think through what to report, and not a *de facto* assessment on the quality of the ethnographic work.

Ethics: Protecting research participants

We close this chapter by commenting on ethics in the sharing of findings from our ethnographic research. Ethnographic research is often focused on a small population or setting. A savvy reader or the person being written about might be able to easily discern who participants are by piecing together information. Therefore, it is essential to find ways to protect participant confidentiality while remaining true to the data. To obscure participants or a setting, we might think about the range of details most relevant to understanding the individual or context. Depending on the study goals and data, this could be location, demographics like gender, ethnicity, or age, or specific events. The research team should consider which details are important to illustrating the central points and which are not. Important details should be included in the end product to help the audience understand key site or participant characteristics.

A few best practices include using general geographic areas such as "Northeast" instead of a specific city, like Boston. Similarly, while it is important to include relevant

Box 5.2 Strategies to protect participants in ethnographic writing

- Use more general geographic areas instead of specific locations such as a city, a specific community, or a named hospital
- Only include general or needed demographic information about study participants
- Do not include quotes with so many details that the speaker could be identified
- Consider developing composite cases

demographic information, such as if a doctor or patient made a particular statement reported in findings, overly specifying who said what could make it easy to identify them. For example, "doctor" might be preferable to "White, female oncologist practicing for >25 years" as the latter might reveal the participant's identity. A good rubric for demographics is to focus on details that are relevant to the research question. For some studies that might be length of time practicing, while for others, it might be gender or race. However, when several details are included, anonymity might be breached.

In the case study to follow, we hear from anthropologist Justeen Hyde about her team's experience in writing up and otherwise disseminating findings from an ethnographic evaluation. Their work reminds us that sharing our findings includes thinking about the audience and the end product(s), and that there are many ways to share pragmatically and ethnographically. Throughout the writing process, it can be helpful to step back and think about practical and actionable takeaways from the data and to consider how refining the formats and/or styles of dissemination can make valuable messages available to a wider audience.

Case 5

Creating space for transparency and dialogue to improve data accuracy and tailored dissemination of ethnographic data

Justeen Hyde

Sometime around 2012, the VA Office of Patient Centred Care and Cultural Transformation (OPCC&CT) set an ambitious goal to radically transform the ways in which health care is conceptualized, organized, delivered, and evaluated in the VA. The transformation is often described as a movement from a biomedical model of care, where the approach is to "find and fix" what is wrong with patients, to one that is focused on whole-person care, which incorporates multiple interconnected domains of life that influence health and well-being (see Figure 5.4). Referred to as Whole Health (National Academies of Sciences 2023), the approach begins with understanding what matters most to each person and providing healthcare that is aligned with their values and preferences. It also includes the use of complementary and integrative health services alongside more conventional ones to expand the range of available treatment options and offers a range of educational and supportive services to help people meet personal health and well-being goals.

In 2016, US Congress passed the Comprehensive Addictions and Recovery Act (CARA), which required VA to reduce opioid prescribing for chronic pain and conduct research to identify and implement nonpharmaceutical treatments for chronic pain and behavioral health problems. Leaders within VA's OPCC&CT seized the opportunity to propel the

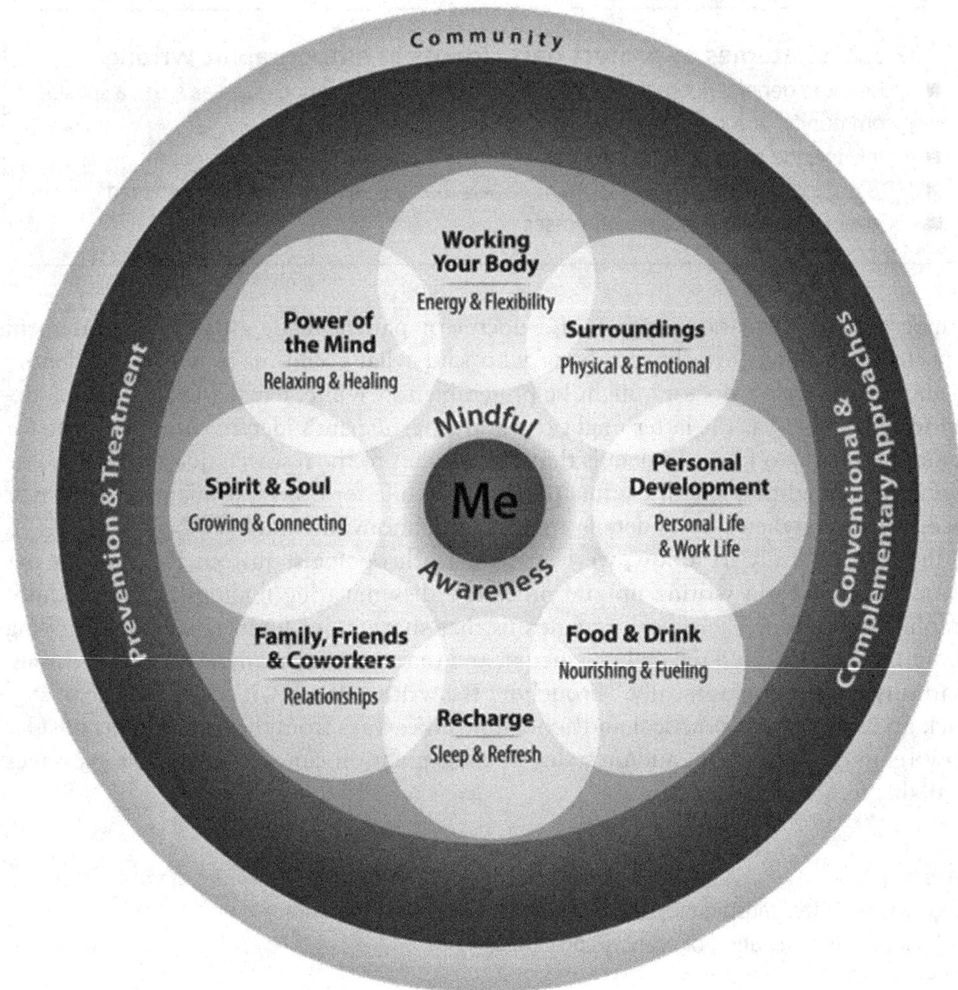

Figure 5.4 VA's conceptual model of Whole Health

Whole Health initiative forward by proposing a full-scale rollout and evaluation of the Whole Health approach in 18 VA medical centers (referred to as Whole Health Flagship Sites). Up until this time there had been some evaluation of different components of Whole Health (see Figure 5.2), but limited guidance existed for medical centers regarding the infrastructure, staffing, and organizational resources needed to make the transformation.

Funding from the CARA legislation supported a large-scale evaluation of implementation and outcomes associated with Whole Health care. Given the nascent guidance for Whole Health implementation at the time and the rapid pace at which details about core components were being developed, the implementation evaluation team wanted a methodological approach that allowed for *learning about* and *learning from* (Savage 2006) Flagship Sites' process, progress, and lessons learned. Ethnographic methods were well-suited to the goals of describing and monitoring the process of change, factors that influenced how sites approached implementation, and evidence of change in clinical practice and organizational priorities. The evaluation team designed a longitudinal,

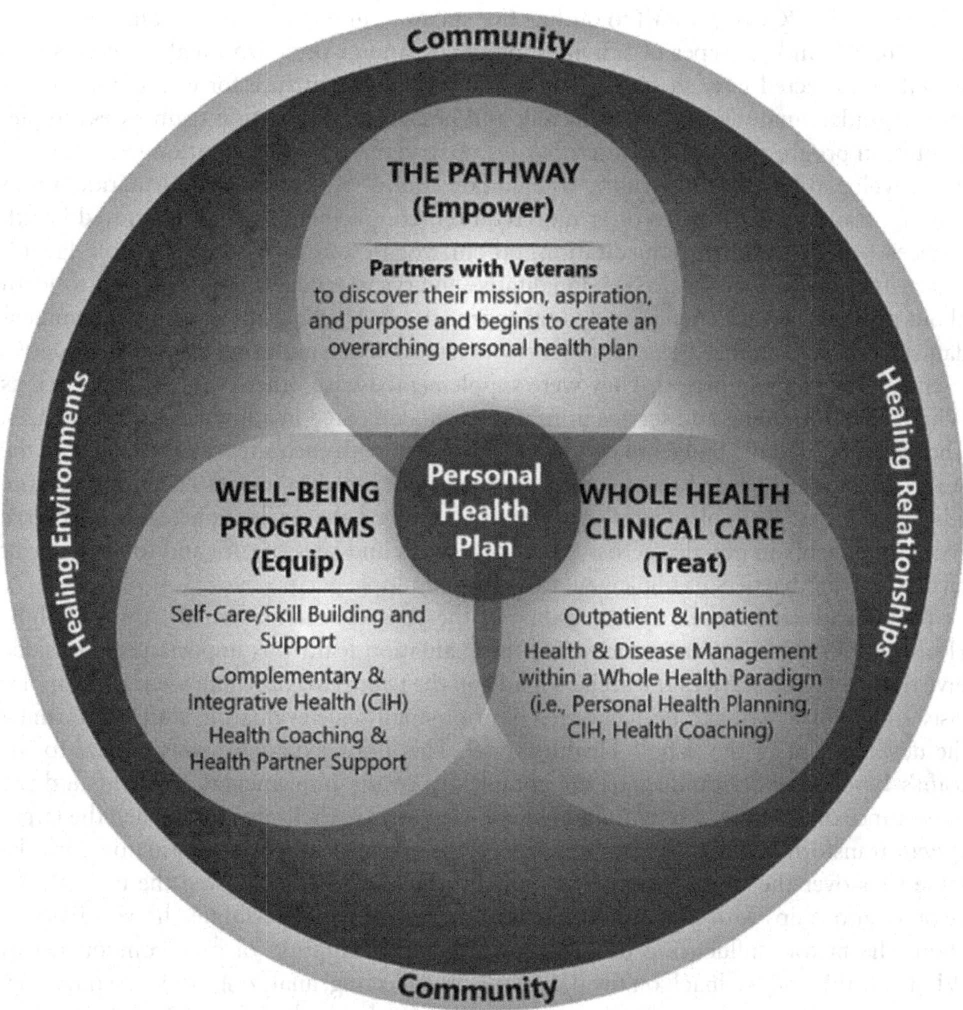

Figure 5.5 Whole Health system of care

mixed-method study with iterative processes of data collection, analysis, reflection, and dissemination to Whole Health leaders involved in implementation at local and national levels. The ethnographic design coupled with a deep commitment to learning from the Flagship sites' experiences allowed the evaluation team and collaborating partners to tack back and forth between theory and practice—between the emerging guidance for how and why to implement core components of Whole Health and what it was like to try and implement in practice. Although measurement of progress toward Whole Health implementation was a goal of the evaluation, the team anticipated that an ethnographic approach would enable continuous reflection on how they were measuring change and inform updates to their approach when differences in theory and practice were observed (Figure 5.5).

The team's first step was to develop a conceptual understanding of the goal for each core component of Whole Health Care and what it would look like in practice (i.e., how would we know the core component is fully implemented). The evaluation team then worked with OPCC&CT staff to outline five stages of implementation (from not started to advanced) and the types of activities, practices, and/or organizational structures that would be expected in each stage. This rubric provided structure for evaluation instruments, guided analysis of data collected, and helped the evaluation team assess implementation progress consistently across sites. A structured implementation tracking tool was developed based on the rubric to facilitate routine collection of information about staffing, training, capacity to offer nine required complementary and integrated health services (e.g., acupuncture, meditation, tai chi, yoga), and provision of Whole Health education and well-being classes. Qualitative interview guides were developed to learn about progress toward change, including approach, successes, challenges, and recommendations. These comprised the core data sources for assessing implementation progress over the 3-year study period. They were supplemented with other types of data, such as Whole Health training and service utilization as documented in administrative databases. The team also had the budget to conduct one site visit with each site over the course of the study, which they decided to use when they assessed a medical center had reached more advanced stages of implementation. Site visits allowed the evaluation team to observe core components in practice across different services and sites of care and to learn about facilitators and barriers to implementation from multiple perspectives.

To cultivate an in-depth understanding of the progress each site made toward Whole Health implementation, the structure of the evaluation team was important to consider. Five trained health services researchers made up the team, two of whom were anthropologists and all of whom had been engaged in prior small-scale evaluation studies informing the development of the Whole Health model. This prior experience was critical to the team's baseline understanding of the complexity of the implementation effort and the importance of developing longitudinal knowledge of how each site approached the larger system transformation. Two team members were assigned to work consistently with the same sites over the study period. This organizational structure allowed the team to develop relationships with site-level Whole Health leaders, which facilitated honest dialogue about the factors influencing progress toward implementation of core components of Whole Health and feedback on the data we were collecting, analyzing, and disseminating.

From the outset, the evaluation team understood the challenges of evaluating an initiative that was "flying as the plane was being built." An ethnographic approach was well-suited for an initiative whose development needed data that could demonstrate accountability and promote continuous learning and development. Weekly meetings were used to critically appraise the quality of the data being used to assess implementation progress, assess consistency in understanding the variability in approach and practice across sites, and talk openly about how each team member's prior experience and perspectives might influence understanding of progress. These deeply reflective conversations were at times challenging on personal levels and for the project. However, they kept the goal of continuous learning and quality improvement at the forefront of the team's work and helped create an openness to feedback from partners when offered.

As a high-profile initiative funded partly through congressional appropriations, data on process and outcomes for each site had both practical and political implications. There were several audiences interested in the data, including local Whole Health and hospital leaders, staff from OPCC&CT (the central office spearheading the transformation), and the US Congress. Findings were also of interest to academic audiences interested in implementation science, healthcare management, and healthcare outcomes, among others. The remainder of this case study highlights how analysis and sharing of evaluation findings contributed to the team's reflexive practice and contributed to the value of the implementation evaluation.

Local Whole Health leaders

The evaluation team decided early in the study to routinely share assessments of progress toward implementation with each site's Whole Health leadership team, which usually consisted of a clinical director, program manager, and local evaluation assistant. People in these roles provided structured qualitative data and the evaluation team wanted to "member check" their summaries with this internal group of key informants before sharing more broadly. Twice a year, brief (~2–3 page) reports summarizing the progress that each site had made toward implementing components of Whole Health care were prepared. Reports highlighted overall progress and progress by core component. A short narrative providing a rationale for the assessment rating of each component was included to allow for transparency in how ratings of progress were derived. This transparency provided a useful way to continuously check the accuracy of the team's understanding of what was happening at each site and obtain feedback on the extent to which the data collected and analyzed were reliably capturing implementation activities. After providing brief reports to local Whole Health leadership teams, the evaluation team requested follow-up conversations (or written communication) to answer questions, further discuss the rationale for ratings, and request input on how to improve data capture. These "member checking" conversations led to modifications in study instruments and deepened understanding of the variety of ways some core components could be implemented.

Conversations about the brief reports highlighted some gaps between theory and practice. For example, a core component of Whole Health care entails engaging veterans in conversations about what matters most in their lives and how their health shapes their ability to engage in meaningful activities. In the original guidance, these conversations were to be initiated by a trained peer or health and wellness coach. Early in the team's data collection, they assumed that if peers and coaches were not yet hired, these conversations were not likely to be happening. What they learned through review and discussion was that there were a variety of different roles assigned to have these conversations; they were taking place, but not necessarily with people in specified roles. This led the evaluation team to discuss the variation in approach with OPCC&CT leads and verify that it could be considered an appropriate way to meet the standard. As a result, the implementation tracking tool was updated to ask about the function of the core component (i.e., conversations about what matters most) in addition to form (i.e., who is having the conversation).

Although transparency in data analysis and reporting had a number of benefits related to continuous learning and improvement in the accuracy of data collection and analysis, it also presented unanticipated challenges and lessons learned. For example, the first brief reports included a bar graph with all 18 sites and their stage of implementation. Each site was given a unique ID, and sites were given their ID only so they see their estimated overall progress on the graph. The evaluation team thought that it would be helpful to know that most sites were in very early stages of implementation and the slow pace of change they were experiencing was common. However, sites began to see themselves as being in competition with each other. Additionally, sites that were at the lowest end of the change spectrum faced questions from their leadership about why they were not advancing at the same rate. This was not the intention of sharing data from all sites. Through ongoing conversations about the "political life" of the data, the team decided to drop the graphic with all sites and reshape the brief reports to only include individual site data.

Office of Patient-Centered Care and Cultural Transformation (OPCC&CT)

Leaders from OPCC&CT espoused a vision of VA as a learning health system, in which information is continuously assessed to feed evaluation, innovation, and improvement. As a result, they valued the routine sharing of data from the 18 Flagship Sites and used the information to improve implementation guidance for local hospitals, workforce trainings, and resources for specific roles (e.g., peer partners). The team knew from prior evaluation work with OPCC&CT that long narrative-style reports were not widely read and brief summary reports or results shared via presentation and slide deck were preferable. Approximately twice a year, they prepared a slide deck highlighting key findings from the implementation study. They presented the data first to people in executive positions (e.g., director, associate director), who often had questions and requested additional information that the team then incorporated (if available). With the updated slide deck, the team then presented to others within OPCC&CT, including regional liaisons and technical assistance providers who could use the information to inform decisions about support provided at the local level.

A key lesson the evaluation team learned from sharing data regularly with their operations partner was related to the language and tone used in the presentation. Changing a large healthcare system is challenging. Much of what they routinely heard about from the sites was about the challenges and factors impeding progress. There were also successes and progress made, but people really wanted to talk about their challenges. The team's first presentation therefore highlighted a long list of challenges that local sites were facing, which they thought would be important for operational partners to hear. On the contrary, they received feedback that the successes, regardless of size, were very important for people to hear too. They also received input on the political nature of some of the challenges raised (e.g., lack of support from hospital leaders) and were encouraged to "flip" the presentation and focus on the "positive deviants" (i.e., the people, contexts, and resources that were successful). The operations partner hoped this would provide people with a better understanding of model approaches to strive for in their work. The team spent hours prior to each report talking about how to carefully navigate the tension between using data to promote change while also calling attention to areas in need of improvement. They developed a structure for reports where equal attention was paid to positive changes and novel practices, as well as opportunities for improvement through additional resources, training, policy, or advocacy.

Congress

With funding for the 18 Flagship Sites coming from congressional appropriation, the implementation team was required to report a variety of findings (e.g., clinical outcomes, patient-reported outcomes) to Congress during the third year of the study (Bokhour et al. 2020). This was a relatively traditional report in many ways and included the rationale for an implementation study, methods, and findings about progress toward implementation. One aspect of the report that was very important to communicate was the enormity of the transformation effort and the length of time it was likely to take to change the culture of and approach to organizing and delivering healthcare services. This important point became clear following the few site visits the team was able to have with more advanced sites prior to the onset of the COVID-19 pandemic. The team realized during these visits that, although sites had accurately reported implementing all of the core Whole Health components, they were not yet at a point of fully integrating these components across different types of services and multiple sites of care. In the report to Congress, the team acknowledged that their implementation study was effective at capturing implementation of core components but that full integration would require different methods and more time to accomplish. They also highlighted systemic changes that needed to be made in order for full integration to happen. At the time of this writing, these changes were still a work in progress.

Conclusions

One of the major challenges of ethnographic research is determining the best ways to share rich and often complex findings with different audiences. The ability to do this well depends to a large extent on understanding the different cultures of each audience, their different values and priorities in relation to the research, the rules of evidence (or what is important to establish credibility), the appropriate language to communicate in, and the most effective formats for communicating findings (e.g., visual, verbal, oral). This case study highlights several ways in which the evaluation team tailored their dissemination strategy and content for different audiences, including the timing of dissemination, the formats in which data were shared, and the amount of data shared at a time. Attention to reflexivity and commitment to transparency enabled the team to continuously learn and improve their evaluation methods. The ethnographic approach was critical to the team's ability to understand and tailor the reporting of data for different audiences, which in turn allowed for complex data to be used to inform and improve efforts to transform healthcare delivery in VA.

References

Addis, Michael E., Wendy A. Wade, and Christina Hatgis. 1999. "Barriers to Dissemination of Evidence-Based Practices: Addressing Practitioners' Concerns about Manual-Based Psychotherapies." *Clinical Psychology: Science and Practice* 6 (4): 430–41. https://doi.org/10.1093/clipsy.6.4.430.

Bokhour, Barbara G., Justeen K. Hyde, Steven Zeliadt, and David C. Mohr. 2020. "Whole Health System of Care Evaluation – A Progress Report on Outcomes of the Whole Health System Pilot at 18 Flagship Sites." White Paper and Interim Report to U.S. Congress.

Buus, Niels, and Amelie Perron. 2020. "The Quality of Quality Criteria: Replicating the Development of the Consolidated Criteria for Reporting Qualitative Research (COREQ)." *International Journal of Nursing Studies* 102 (February): 103452. https://doi.org/10.1016/j.ijnurstu.2019.103452.

Cahill, Mairead, Katie Robinson, Judith Pettigrew, Rose Galvin, and Mandy Stanley. 2018. "Qualitative Synthesis: A Guide to Conducting a Meta-Ethnography." *British Journal of Occupational Therapy* 81 (3): 129–37. https://doi.org/10.1177/0308022617745016.

Clark, Alexander M., and David R. Thompson. 2016. "Five Tips for Writing Qualitative Research in High-Impact Journals: Moving From #BMJnoQual." *International Journal of Qualitative Methods* 15 (1): 160940691664125. https://doi.org/10.1177/1609406916641250.

Creese, Jennifer, John-Paul Byrne, Rebecca Olson, and Niamh Humphries. 2023. "A Catalyst for Change: Developing a Collaborative Reflexive Ethnographic Approach to Research with Hospital Doctors during the COVID-19 Pandemic." *Methodological Innovations* 16 (1): 3–14. https://doi.org/10.1177/20597991221137813.

Cunningham-Erves, Jennifer, Tilicia Mayo-Gamble, Yolanda Vaughn, Jim Hawk, Mike Helms, Claudia Barajas, and Yvonne Joosten. 2020. "Engagement of Community Stakeholders to Develop a Framework to Guide Research Dissemination to Communities." *Health Expectations* 23 (4): 958–68. https://doi.org/10.1111/hex.13076.

Dyer, Karen E., Sharyn J. Potter, Alison B. Hamilton, Tana M. Luger, Alicia A. Bergman, Elizabeth M. Yano, and Ruth Klap. 2019. "Gender Differences in Veterans' Perceptions of Harassment on Veterans Health Administration Grounds." *Women's Health Issues* 29 (June): S83–93. https://doi.org/10.1016/j.whi.2019.04.016.

Fenwick, Karissa M., Rachel E. Golden, Susan M. Frayne, Alison B. Hamilton, Elizabeth M. Yano, Diane V. Carney, and Ruth Klap. 2021. "Women Veterans' Experiences of Harassment and Perceptions of Veterans Affairs Health Care Settings during a National Anti-Harassment Campaign." *Women's Health Issues* 31 (6): 567–75. https://doi.org/10.1016/j.whi.2021.06.005.

Fenwick, Karissa M., Sharyn J. Potter, Ruth Klap, Karen E. Dyer, Mark R. Relyea, Elizabeth M. Yano, Tana M. Luger, Alicia A. Bergman, Joya G. Chrystal, and Alison B. Hamilton. 2021. "Staff and Patient Perspectives on Bystander Intervention Training to Address Patient-Initiated Sexual Harassment in Veterans Affairs Healthcare Settings." *Women's Health Issues* 31 (6): 576–85. https://doi.org/10.1016/j.whi.2021.07.003.

Fix, Gemmae M., Trenton M. Haltom, Alison M. Cogan, Stephanie L. Shimada, and Jessica A. Davila. 2023. "Understanding Patients' Preferences and Experiences during an Electronic Health Record Transition." *Journal of General Internal Medicine*, August. https://doi.org/10.1007/s11606-023-08338-6.

Fix, Gemmae M., Justeen K. Hyde, Rendelle E. Bolton, Victoria A. Parker, Kelly Dvorin, Juliet Wu, Avy A. Skolnik, et al. 2018. "The Moral Discourse of HIV Providers within Their Organizational Context: An Ethnographic Case Study." *Patient Education and Counseling* 101 (12): 2226–32. https://doi.org/10.1016/j.pec.2018.08.018.

Glasgow, Russell E. 2013. "What Does It Mean to Be Pragmatic? Pragmatic Methods, Measures, and Models to Facilitate Research Translation." *Health Education & Behavior* 40 (3): 257–65. https://doi.org/10.1177/1090198113486805.

Greenhalgh, Trisha, Ellen Annandale, Richard Ashcroft, James Barlow, Nick Black, Alan Bleakley, Ruth Boaden, et al. 2016. "An Open Letter to *The BMJ* Editors on Qualitative Research." *BMJ*, 352: i563. https://doi.org/10.1136/bmj.i563.

Hamilton, Alison. 2013. "Qualitative Methods in Rapid Turn-around Health Services Research." VA HSR&D Cyberseminar Spotlight on Women's Health, December 11. http://www.hsrd.research.va.gov/for_researchers/cyber_seminars/archives/780-notes.pdf.

Jackson, George L., Benjamin J. Powers, Ranee Chatterjee, Janet Prvu Bettger, Alex R. Kemper, Vic Hasselblad, Rowena J. Dolor, et al. 2013. "The Patient-Centered Medical Home: A Systematic Review." *Annals of Internal Medicine* 158 (3): 169. https://doi.org/10.7326/0003-4819-158-3-201302050-00579.

Klap, Ruth, Jill E. Darling, Alison B. Hamilton, Danielle E. Rose, Karen Dyer, Ismelda Canelo, Sally Haskell, and Elizabeth M. Yano. 2019. "Prevalence of Stranger Harassment of Women Veterans at Veterans Affairs Medical Centers and Impacts on Delayed and Missed Care." *Women's Health Issues* 29 (2): 107–15. https://doi.org/10.1016/j.whi.2018.12.002.

Lincoln, Yvonna S., and Egon G. Guba. 1985. *Naturalistic Inquiry*. Beverly Hills, CA: Sage Publications.

Montagnes, David J. S., E. Ian Montagnes, and Zhou Yang. 2022. "Finding Your Scientific Story by Writing Backwards." *Marine Life Science & Technology* 4 (1): 1–9. https://doi.org/10.1007/s42995-021-00120-z.

Morse, Jan M., Michael Barrett, Maria Mayan, Karin Olson, and Jude Spiers. 2002. "Verification Strategies for Establishing Reliability and Validity in Qualitative Research." *International Journal of Qualitative Methods* 1 (2): 13–22.

National Academies of Sciences. 2023. *Achieving Whole Health: A New Approach for Veterans and the Nation*. Washington, D.C: The National Academies Press.

O'Brien, Bridget C., Ilene B. Harris, Thomas J. Beckman, Darcy A. Reed, and David A. Cook. 2014. "Standards for Reporting Qualitative Research: A Synthesis of Recommendations." *Academic Medicine* 89 (9): 1245–51. https://doi.org/10.1097/ACM.0000000000000388.

Obert, Jeanne L., Alison Hamilton Brown, Joan Zweben, Darrell Christian, Jenn Delmhorst, Sam Minsky, Patrick Morrisey, Denna Vandersloot, and Ahndrea Weiner. 2005. "When Treatment Meets Research: Clinical Perspectives from the CSAT Methamphetamine Treatment Project." *Journal of Substance Abuse Treatment* 28 (3): 231–37. https://doi.org/10.1016/j.jsat.2004.12.008.

Patton, Michael Quinn. 2003. "Qualitative Evaluation Checklist." September 2003. https://wmich.edu/sites/default/files/attachments/u350/2014/qualitativeevalchecklist.pdf.

Savage, Jan. 2006. "Ethnographic Evidence: The Value of Applied Ethnography in Healthcare." *Journal of Research in Nursing* 11 (5): 383–93. https://doi.org/10.1177/1744987106068297.

Schindler, Larissa, and Hilmar Schäfer. 2021. "Practices of Writing in Ethnographic Work." *Journal of Contemporary Ethnography* 50 (1): 11–32. https://doi.org/10.1177/0891241620923396.

Solimeo, Samantha L., Sarah S. Ono, Kenda R. Stewart, Michelle A. Lampman, Gary E. Rosenthal, and Greg L. Stewart. 2017. "Gatekeepers as Care Providers: The Care Work of Patient-centered Medical Home Clerical Staff." *Medical Anthropology Quarterly* 31 (1): 97–114. https://doi.org/10.1111/maq.12281.

Solimeo, Samantha L., Greg L. Stewart, and Gary E. Rosenthal. 2016. "The Critical Role of Clerks in the Patient-Centered Medical Home." *The Annals of Family Medicine* 14 (4): 377–79. https://doi.org/10.1370/afm.1934.

Stange, Kurt C. 2006. "Publishing Multimethod Research." *The Annals of Family Medicine* 4 (4): 292–94. https://doi.org/10.1370/afm.615.

Timmermans, Stefan. 2012. "How to Get Published in Social Science & Medicine? An Editorial from the Medical Sociology Office." September 3, 2012. https://www.sciencedirect.com/journal/social-science-and-medicine/about/policies.

Tong, Allison, Peter Sainsbury, and Jonathan Craig. 2007. "Consolidated Criteria for Reporting Qualitative Research (COREQ): A 32-Item Checklist for Interviews and Focus Groups." *International Journal for Quality in Health Care* 19 (6): 349–57. https://doi.org/10.1093/intqhc/mzm042.

CHAPTER 6

Crafting a new ethnography

Introduction

Chapters and case studies in this book build on an exciting moment in healthcare research, as ethnographic approaches are increasingly recognized for their value in helping to better understand the complex work and dynamic relationships of healthcare (Waring, Marshall, and Bishop 2015). In this closing chapter, we consider ethnographic innovations emerging in healthcare research, how many of these innovations are feeding back into the social sciences, and how ethnography can support learning healthcare systems in a rapidly shifting social and technological world.

New opportunities for ethnographic theory and methods

Throughout this book, we highlight how pragmatic healthcare ethnography prioritizes lived experience and cultural relativity, seeks to develop holistic understandings of complex problems, engages with reflexivity and power, and responds flexibly to the challenges of working in dynamic environments and amid emergent and often unexpected findings. Over the past few decades, the early tropes of the lone ethnographer dutifully observing and interpreting have given way to what Creese and colleagues (2023) have called the "new ethnographic ideals" of "collaboration, reflexivity, and impact." These new ideals, in turn, have catalyzed innovations in ethnographic theory and methods, with broad potential for application and impact.

In one example of such innovations, Creese's own team (2023) developed a method for conducting ethnography during the COVID-19 pandemic that precluded on-site observation in most healthcare settings. They sought to better understand experiences of frontline healthcare work and burnout among physicians in Ireland and drew upon regular text exchanges via WhatsApp as a primary source of data collection. This strategy required physicians to engage in recurrent communication and reporting, but also in concerted reflection. Writing up the study, the authors argued this mobile instant messaging ethnography, while reliant upon a highly lean form of communication (i.e.,

DOI: 10.4324/9781003390657-6

texting), achieved core elements of an ethnographic approach, including "emic perspective, engagement, flexibility, contextualization and description-based analysis." By creating opportunities for dialogue and data collection when participants were at home as well as in the hospital, the researchers were able to observe how participants were thinking about, recovering from, and preparing for work in their homes. This approach not only integrated the collaborative engagement and ongoing interactions of longitudinal ethnography but also was able to capture insights that may have remained invisible in hospital-based observation.

In another innovative example, a co-designed partnership research program in Australia used focused ethnography to examine implementation of an electronic information management system across local health districts (Conte et al. 2019). A core team of ethnographers engaged in intensive visits at each of 14 sites, capturing data using ethnographic fieldnotes, pictures, and recordings in ways that allowed for ongoing and retroactive analysis. Early findings and preliminary analyses were shared with research participants and partners. The team identified how formal implementation of the information system was accompanied by a proliferation of informal strategies for working with the system, via spreadsheets, tip sheets, and other tools. The authors found that collecting and revisiting these data with research partners "extended the ethnographic 'place'" and prompted "ongoing consideration of our role, perspectives on the data, and our ability to facilitate change through the research process." Not only were their collaborative and reflexive methods successful in revealing the implementation challenges and creative adaptations occurring at sites, but the resulting discussions prompted reconsideration of the larger program and how its goals for future expansion might be updated.

Ethnographic theory has benefited from this turn toward the reflexive, and not only in the context of healthcare. Shattuck and colleagues (2022) conducted five years of ethnographic work as part of an implementation trial to improve the social safety and reduce minority stress of LGBTQ+ students in New Mexico schools. Integrating findings from individual and small-group interviews and periodic reflections, they demonstrate the myriad ways in which implementation teams in each school tried to work with (and sometimes against) school hierarchies to leverage power and support improvements for LGBTQ+ students. They conclude ultimately that efforts toward implementation and improvement "must attend to the multiple real and perceived power structures that shape implementation environments and influence organizational readiness and individual motivation." Similarly, Snell-Rood and colleagues (2021) have pointed to the relevance of critical theories—theories that consider how structural (e.g., social, cultural, or economic) factors impact individual and population well-being—in implementation science, particularly in efforts to address health equity.

Each of these studies provides an example of how complex, fully realized ethnography is occurring in contemporary health research, and evolving the field in doing so. This expanding ethnographic range is feeding back into the social science disciplines in a kind of "cross-pollination" (Black et al. 2021), encouraging greater transparency in methods and reporting, more active engagement of and agency for partners in collaborative research, and enhanced relevance and impact in the conduct and dissemination of ethnographic work (Closser and Finley 2016). Traditional standards for communicating findings in the academic social sciences—reading carefully composed papers at conferences, writing and speaking in specialist jargon, and offering minimal detail on methods for data collection and analysis—face increasing pushback in more applied settings. The growing availability of anthropology, sociology, business, and other programs offering advanced training in applied ethnographic methods has fostered novel approaches to teaching ethnographic theory and methods (Hayes and Jung 2023; McGranahan 2018). Meanwhile, shifting job markets have resulted in a greater presence of anthropologists on multidisciplinary research teams (Fix et al. 2023), and the integration of social scientists and now social science methods into healthcare's most wicked problems allows for an opportunity to develop "wicked scientists" (Kawa et al. 2021). Given the rate of emerging progress, this book may be less a summary of ethnographic how-to and more a glimpse into the ethnographic future.

Ethnography as part of learning healthcare systems

Ethnography may also bring unlooked-for insights as a way of approaching health and healthcare. A recent scoping review went so far as to argue that engaging in ethnography can encourage ongoing healthcare improvement because "the ethnographic paradigm can encourage good habits (resilience, creativity, learning, systems thinking and influencing)" as well as "reflection, problem-finding, and exposing hidden practices" (Black et al. 2021). Ethnography can be most valuable precisely where it helps us to see the unconsidered and unexpected. In their article on the oscillation between ethnographic theory and practice, Cubellis, Schmid, and von Peter (2021) reported on a comparison of two financial models for psychiatric care in Germany, a fee-for-service model and a capitation model offering a fixed budget based on the number of service users. What emerged from the analysis was not a difference in the care associated with the financial models themselves, but the drain on time and resources for care delivery associated with clinic inspections required under the fee-for-service model. It was not the financing of care that made a difference, but rather the unequal administrative load associated with the fee-for-service model that impacted providers' ability to deliver timely and effective care.

Given all this, it is perhaps no surprise that ethnography has come of age in healthcare research alongside the idea of a learning health system, defined as a "system in which science, informatics, incentives, and culture are aligned for continuous improvement and innovation" (Smith and Institute of Medicine (US) 2013). The notion of continuous informational and relational feedback loops is inherent to a learning health system. It aligns beautifully with the examples of ethnographic practice seen throughout this book, in which providers function as ethnographers, veterans and family members and community partners participate actively in defining and developing knowledge and action goals, problems are identified and explored, and novel solutions are tried, examined, and refined. As Gala True described in reflecting on her case study (see Chapter 3) of working with community members to reduce firearm suicides among veterans, there was a "cyclical nature" to the work:

> … where ethnographic work helps build a foundation of understanding and shared goals, which then leads to reciprocity whereby the community partners help the health researchers and the health researchers do what they can to address the concerns of community partners, which then leads to deeper trust and sustained collaboration….

For Alison, Gemmae, and Erin, as researchers embedded within the VA as a learning health system, we are constantly trying to foster increasing connectedness, creativity, and systems thinking, as well as co-learning and high-impact problem-solving. A pragmatic ethnographic approach remains an essential, and increasingly prominent, part of this work.

References

Black, Georgia B., Sandra Van Os, Samantha Machen, and Naomi J. Fulop. 2021. "Ethnographic Research as an Evolving Method for Supporting Healthcare Improvement Skills: A Scoping Review." *BMC Medical Research Methodology* 21 (1): 274. https://doi.org/10.1186/s12874-021-01466-9.

Closser, Svea, and Erin P. Finley. 2016. "A New Reflexivity: Why Anthropology Matters in Contemporary Health Research and Practice, and How to Make It Matter More: A New Reflexivity." *American Anthropologist* 118 (2): 385–90. https://doi.org/10.1111/aman.12532.

Conte, Kathleen P., Abeera Shahid, Sisse Grøn, Victoria Loblay, Amanda Green, Christine Innes-Hughes, Andrew Milat, et al. 2019. "Capturing Implementation Knowledge: Applying Focused Ethnography to Study How Implementers Generate and Manage Knowledge in the Scale-up of Obesity Prevention Programs." *Implementation Science* 14 (1): 91. https://doi.org/10.1186/s13012-019-0938-7.

Creese, Jennifer, John-Paul Byrne, Rebecca Olson, and Niamh Humphries. 2023. "A Catalyst for Change: Developing a Collaborative Reflexive Ethnographic Approach to Research with Hospital Doctors during the COVID-19 Pandemic." *Methodological Innovations* 16 (1): 3–14. https://doi.org/10.1177/20597991221137813.

Cubellis, Lauren, Christine Schmid, and Sebastian Von Peter. 2021. "Ethnography in Health Services Research: Oscillation between Theory and Practice." *Qualitative Health Research* 31 (11): 2029–40. https://doi.org/10.1177/10497323211022312.

Fix, Gemmae, Aaron Seaman, Linda Nichols, Sarah Ono, Nicholas Rattray, Samantha Solimeo, Heather Schacht Reisinger, and Traci Abraham. 2023. "Building a Community of Anthropological Practice: The Case of Anthropologists Working within the United States' Largest Health Care System." *Human Organization* 82 (2): 169–81. https://doi.org/10.17730/1938-3525-82.2.169.

Hayes, Lauren, and Yuson Jung. 2023. "Beyond Methods: A Model for Teaching Theory in Applied Anthropology." *Annals of Anthropological Practice* 47 (1): 20–34. https://doi.org/10.1111/napa.12194.

Kawa, Nicholas C., Mark Anthony Arceño, Ryan Goeckner, Chelsea E. Hunter, Steven J. Rhue, Shane A. Scaggs, Matthew E. Biwer, et al. 2021. "Training Wicked Scientists for a World of Wicked Problems." *Humanities and Social Sciences Communications* 8 (1): 189. https://doi.org/10.1057/s41599-021-00871-1.

McGranahan, Carole. 2018. "Ethnography beyond Method: The Importance of an Ethnographic Sensibility." *Sites: A Journal of Social Anthropology and Cultural Studies* 15 (1). https://doi.org/10.11157/sites-id373.

Shattuck, Daniel, Bonnie O. Richard, Elise Trott Jaramillo, Evelyn Byrd, and Cathleen E. Willging. 2022. "Power and Resistance in Schools: Implementing Institutional Change to Promote Health Equity for Sexual and Gender Minority Youth." *Frontiers in Health Services* 2 (November): 920790. https://doi.org/10.3389/frhs.2022.920790.

Smith, Mark D., and Institute of Medicine (US), eds. 2013. *Best Care at Lower Cost: The Path to Continuously Learning Health Care in America*. Washington, D.C.: National Academies Press.

Snell-Rood, Claire, Elise Trott Jaramillo, Alison B. Hamilton, Sarah E. Raskin, Francesca M. Nicosia, and Cathleen Willging. 2021. "Advancing Health Equity through a Theoretically Critical Implementation Science." *Translational Behavioral Medicine* 11 (8): 1617–25. https://doi.org/10.1093/tbm/ibab008.

Waring, Justin, Fiona Marshall, and Simon Bishop. 2015. "Understanding the Occupational and Organizational Boundaries to Safe Hospital Discharge." *Journal of Health Services Research and Policy* 20 (1_suppl): 35–44. https://doi.org/10.1177/1355819614552512.

Afterword

Annette Boaz, PhD

As an undergraduate and postgraduate student, I was impressed by the work of anthropologists and the depth of insight generated by their immersive studies. I can still visualize the Balinese cockfights described by Clifford Geertz (1973) and the ways in which he used these spectacles to provide rich insights into Balinese society and culture.

Anthropological accounts, typically written following long periods of time spent with distant communities, have captured the imagination of generations of researchers, including my own. Twenty years ago, I began thinking about the potential for using ethnographic methods in my own work in healthcare research. In particular, I was inspired by Julia Lawton's ethnographic study of palliative care, which challenged conventional ideas of death and dying through a nuanced account of patient experiences of hospice care (Lawton 2000).

Before I had a go at conducting ethnographic research, I had a little preview of what observations could bring to my understanding of a subject. At the time we were collecting data for a study looking at healthy eating in primary schools. The children had been given an intervention (a colorful fridge chart) to encourage them to eat more fruit and vegetables. We brought the children together in focus groups to tell us how it had gone. The children began to share enthusiastic accounts of their fruit and vegetable eating until one little girl pointed out that she had seen another member of the group eating cookies earlier that day. Her observation sent the conversation off in a completely different direction. The boy held his head in his hands and explained how hard it was to change habits. The others nodded in agreement and offered him their support and sympathy! It made me think about what I might learn if I employed the power of observation in my applied healthcare research.

In subsequent years, I have often found that insights from time spent in the field have not only generated insights in their own right but have also enhanced other methods. For example, shared experience and understanding (and trust) generated by time in the field can generate rich accounts of patient, carer, and staff experience in semi-structured interviews, as Alison, Gemmae, and Erin describe in Chapter 3.

When I tried out ethnography myself, I was struck by the additional understanding I gained from spending time in a setting, getting to know people and processes in context. However, as an applied health services researcher, the length of time needed to conduct ethnographic studies felt like a major barrier to using the approach. The idea that the researcher might spend long periods of time conducting observations felt at odds with the conventional practices of health services research. Was there really time and resources available to 'hang around'? In one of my studies, we found that limitations of observational time could be overcome by making the most of observational periods, situating quality improvement efforts within the clinical practice context, achieving "attunement" with local clinical cultures, and engaging participants in guiding study design (Vougioukalou et al. 2019). What is encouraging about this book is that it makes such a strong case for ethnography in applied healthcare research. It uses examples throughout to illustrate how ethnography can be used as a practical approach in the healthcare researcher's methodological toolbox, with particular insights from the US Veterans Health Administration, which has long led the way in reforming the practice of research.

I am especially impressed by the case made in this book for ethnography as an approach that helps us address the challenges we face in studying the complexities of modern healthcare systems. Alison, Erin, and Gemmae and their contributing colleagues highlight the holistic nature of ethnography and its flexibility—both powerful factors in designing applied healthcare research. Ethnography helps to address a number of the critiques of research practice. First, it brings lived experience to the center of the research enterprise (Boulton and Boaz 2019). Second, it deals with the critical issue of power (O'Shea, Boaz, and Chambers 2019). Finally, ethnography requires a high level of reflexivity. The role of the researcher and their relationship to the topic, the context, and the actors form a key part of written accounts of ethnography—the ethnographer is never 'written out' of the research account.

Ethnography brings with it interesting challenges, as researchers seek to spend time in healthcare settings without getting in the way. I have been fortunate to have doctoral students who used ethnographic methods in their PhD research, made possible by the longer timelines of a typical PhD course of study. I remember discussing with one of my students how she might make herself useful in her study setting (by making tea or answering the phone) without compromising her ethnographic work. Another PhD student with a clinical background wanted to wear her uniform while spending time conducting ethnographic research on a busy maternity ward. She felt this would help her blend into the setting. However, the reassuring presence of a uniform in the room meant that the staff on duty felt they could safely leave the patient and my student ended up catching the newborn baby! After that, she dressed in her own clothes to reinforce to staff that she was not an extra pair of clinical hands.

These accounts are potentially impactful in that they can shift thinking, helping us to re-evaluate what we know and what to think differently about the health and social care challenges we face. I love the examples in Chapter 6 of ethnographers innovating to continue to conduct ethnographic work in the pandemic. For example, Creese and colleagues (2023) managed to maintain core elements of an ethnographic approach by substituting on-site observation text exchanges via WhatsApp to look at burnout in the healthcare workforce. I was in a similar situation, where my role in the field was picked up by clinical colleagues who trained up to conduct observations and informal interviews and joined me for weekly check-in calls to discuss what they were seeing and learning.

As with the classic ethnographies, the golden nuggets in this book are the accounts of ethnographic practice shared by the authors. However, there is also a lot of helpful information for anyone interested in exploring the potential contribution of pragmatic healthcare ethnography. I can see this book being of use to students, researchers of all levels, and clinical academics. Hopefully it will go some way to adding ethnography into the toolbox of applied healthcare researchers of the future, ensuring that rich ethnographic insights into what we actually do (as opposed to what we think we do or hope we do) can play a more central role in health care and outcomes (Boaz et al. 2016). Reading the book has inspired me to think again about ethnography in my next study and I look forward to sharing the book with friends and colleagues.

References

Boaz, Annette, Glenn Robert, Louise Locock, Gordon Sturmey, Melanie Gager, Sofia Vougioukalou, Sue Ziebland, and Jonathan Fielden. 2016. "What Patients Do and Their Impact on Implementation: An Ethnographic Study of Participatory Quality Improvement Projects in English Acute Hospitals." Edited by Aoife M. McDermottand Anne Reff Pedersen. *Journal of Health Organization and Management* 30 (2): 258–78. https://doi.org/10.1108/JHOM-02-2015-0027.

Boulton, Richard, and Annette Boaz. 2019. "The Emotional Labour of Quality Improvement Work in End of Life Care: A Qualitative Study of Patient and Family Centred Care (PFCC) in England." *BMC Health Services Research* 19 (1): 923. https://doi.org/10.1186/s12913-019-4762-1.

Creese, Jennifer, John-Paul Byrne, Rebecca Olson, and Niamh Humphries. 2023. "A Catalyst for Change: Developing a Collaborative Reflexive Ethnographic Approach to Research with Hospital Doctors during the COVID-19 Pandemic." *Methodological Innovations* 16 (1): 3–14. https://doi.org/10.1177/20597991221137813.

Geertz, Clifford. 1973. *The Interpretation of Cultures*. New York, New York: Basic Books.

Lawton, Julia. 2000. *The Dying Process: Patients' Experiences of Palliative Care*. London; New York: Routledge.

O'Shea, Alison, Annette L. Boaz, and Mary Chambers. 2019. "A Hierarchy of Power: The Place of Patient and Public Involvement in Healthcare Service Development." *Frontiers in Sociology* 4 (May): 38. https://doi.org/10.3389/fsoc.2019.00038.

Vougioukalou, Sofia, Annette Boaz, Melanie Gager, and Louise Locock. 2019. "The Contribution of Ethnography to the Evaluation of Quality Improvement in Hospital Settings: Reflections on Observing Co-Design in Intensive Care Units and Lung Cancer Pathways in the UK." *Anthropology & Medicine* 26 (1): 18–32. https://doi.org/10.1080/13648470.2018.1507104.

Index

Note: Page numbers in **bold** and *italics* refer to tables and figures, respectively.

accessibility 16–17
Agar, Michael 52
Aijazi, Omer 44
analytic templates 81–85
applied ethnography 5
approvals **16**, 17, 28–33
Atkins, David xviii, 89

bi-directional communication 43
Bikker, A. P. 56–57
bio-cultural model of health 15
Blackwell, Gretta 52
Bond, Virginia 58
Brunner, Julian 82
Bunce, Arwen E. 55, 57, 73

Chasing Polio in Pakistan (Closser) 103
Closser, Svea 55, 103
codes/coding 73, 77, 80, 85–88, 91, 97
Consolidated Criteria for Reporting Qualitative Research (COREQ) 108
COVID-19 pandemic 33–35, 58, 115, 119
credibility 43–45, 62, 64–65, 107, 115
Creese, Jennifer 119
3 Cs (context, content, concepts) of observation 47
Cubellis, Lauren 121
cultural relativism 10

data analysis 18, 59, 63, 67, 74, *74*, 113; familiarization 75–76; organizational system for analysis 75; pragmatic 73; procedure 89; qualitative 74–75, 83, 88; strategic 76–77; and understanding *74*
data collection 1–4, 8, 15, 18, **20**, 23, 28, 31–32, 41, 43, 46, 56–57, 61, 63, 74–80, 88, 98, 111, 113, 119–120; episodes 65, 80; ethnographic 55, 59; events 65; semi structured 83, smartphone-enabled 51; structured 47, 67; team 74; tools 47; unstructured 67
data familiarization 75–76, 87, 97
data summary 21–23, **23**
diagramming 81–85, 97
document/archival review **18**, 19

electronic health record (EHR) 104
Eliacin, Johanne xix
emergence 4, 78, *78*
emic 2, 7, 10, **34**, 51, 55, 87, 92, 120
episode profiles memos 78, 79–80
epistemology 6–7, 9–11
ethnography: defining 1–2; design 17; epistemology in RAP 10–11; epistemology of 7; features 34; flexibility 4; gatekeepers 28; inherently holistic 3–4; lived experiences 3; methodological fit 6; methods in healthcare environments 6; methods in studies **18**; overview 1–2, 6;

participants in research 30; power, concerned with 4; questions to consider **16**; reflexivity 4; strategies to protect participants 109; themes of 2–4; as tool for change 7–10; writing 100

Facundo, Ray 64–65
familiarization 75; *see also* data familiarization
feasibility 5, 15–17, 23, 28, 51, 67, 107
Fereday, Jennifer 87
Fetters, Michael D. 46
fieldnotes 10, 25, 34–36, 41, 46–50, 52, 55, 61, 67, 73, 75–77, 81, 83, 99, 107, 120; unstructured 46–48
Fields of Combat (Erin) 103
findings, ethnographic 97–99; audiences and common products **104**; data sources and analytic resources 99–100; journals and publishing ethnographic work 100–103, 114; local whole health leaders 113–114; nonacademic products 103–106; sharing 97–98, *98*
focused ethnography 5, 45–46, 120
focus groups **18**, 19, 52
Fortney, John 8
Fresquez, Sari 63

Google Sheets 83
Greenhalgh, Trisha 3, 59, 88, 101

healthcare research, ethnography for 15; appropriateness 15–17; approvals 28–33; goal 21–22, **21–22**; planning 20–23, **21**; sampling 23–28; study design 18–20
Hinder, Susan 3
Hyde, Justeen xix, 50, 109–113

Illness Narratives, The (Kleinman) 103
individual interviews 17–18, **18**, 42–43, 98, 120
infographics 66, 104–105
institutional review board (IRB) 28–29; protocol 62; strategies to get ethnographic study approved by 29; study protocol describing observation 30–31
integrated mixed-method approach 55
International Journal of Qualitative Methods 101
interviews 1–18, 28, 50–62, 83–84, 87–88, 125; brief 20; features of 50; focus groups 52; formal 46; guide 35, 77; individual 17–18, **18**, 42–43, 98, 120; layering 36; one-time 50–51; patient and provider interviews 52–53; periodic reflections 53–55; qualitative 44, 106, 112; rapid qualitative interviews 51–52; scheduling 19; semi-structured **26**, **34**, 42; telephone or in-person 32; transcripts 76; unstructured 76, 79

Journal Author Name Estimator (JANE) website 101
Journal of Ethnicity in Substance Abuse 79
Journal of General Internal Medicine 106

Kara, Hanna 52
Kleinman, Arthur 37, 103
Kroeger, Karen A. 58

MacDonald, James 52
Maietta, Ray xxi
McCullough, Megan 33–38, 88, 100
McGranahan, Carole 50
Medical Anthropology Quarterly 101
memoing 77–80, 97; emergent discoveries memo 78, **78**; episode profiles **78**, 79–80; future studies 78, **78**; methods 77, **78**; project-level memo templates 75; research question 77–78, **78**; topic memos **78**, 80
methodology/methodological: approach 41, 90, 92; challenges 59; coherence 18, 89, 108; fit 6; innovations 6; orientation 108; pluralism 73; structured 58; toolbox 124
Microsoft Excel 83
Microsoft PowerPoint 82–83
Microsoft Word 83
mixed-methods 74; analysis 82–83; joint displays 82; studies 101
Moeckli, Jane 9
Morse, Janice M. 89, 108
Muir-Cochrane, Eimear 87

observation 3, 15, **18**, 19–20, **20**, 28, 30, **34**, 44–50, 64–65, 77, 80, 90, 99, 107; clinic 1–2; 3 Cs (context, content, concepts) 47; data collection 31; direct 3; fieldnotes and other methods of documenting 46–48; IRB study protocol and 30–31; non-participant 42, 45; on-site 54; participant 3, 45; reflexive 60
online ethnography 58
online methods 58
Ono, Sarah 90–92
on-site observation 54

PACT (Patient-Aligned Care Teams) 90–91
Palinkas, Lawrence A. 73
participants 7, 17, **20**, 22, 27–29, 34, 44, 50–52, 60–63, 83, 88–92, 99, 120, 124; in ethnographic research 30–31; experiences of 43; materials 60; protecting 108–109; recruiting 119
participatory action research (PAR) 63
patient advisory groups *105*
Patton, Michael Quinn 108
periodic reflections 53–55
photovoice methods 64
podcasts 106

Pomales, Tony 34
post-traumatic stress disorder (PTSD) 41, 100; veterans with 7–8, 17, 41
power 43–44; dynamics 4
pragmatic ethnography 41–43, 73; data analysis 73; features of 89; focus groups 52; interviews 50–52; knowledge and expertise 53; observation 44–50; participatory approaches 59–68; patient and provider interviews 52–53; periodic reflections 53–55; power 43–44; rapid, virtual, online, and video ethnographic approaches 57–59; reflexivity 43–44; rigor, trustworthiness, and constraint 59; team-based ethnography 55–57; trust 43–44
pragmatism 5–6
project manager **56**
Proudfoot, Kevin 87

Quality Enhancement Research Initiative (QUERI) program xix
quality improvement (QI) 29, 112, 124
quantitative studies 16, **22**, 23, 27, 34, 44, 73, 82, 87–88, 91, 101; data analysis software 75; data collection spectrum *76*; guides 112

randomized controlled trial 8
Rapid Assessment Procedure-Informed Clinical Ethnography (RAPICE) 73
Rapid Assessment Process (RAP) 8–9; ethnographic epistemology 10–11
reflexivity 43–44
Reisinger, Heather Schacht 6–7, 9–10, 82
research questions, ethnographic case studies **16**, 16–17; accessibility **16**; approvals **16**; frequency **16**; suitability **16**
rigor 6, 9, 41, 49, 55–57, 59, 74, 77, 88–89, 104, 106–108
risks minimization to participants 31
risks to participants or research team 32
Rubinstein, Ellen B. 47

sample analytic synthesis template 84
Sangaramoorthy, Thurka 58
Schmid, Christine 121
semi-structured: fieldnote 47–48, 51; interviews **26**, **34**, 35, 79, 124; qualitative data 83
sensibility, ethnographic 50
setbacks, dealing with 32–33
Shattuck, Daniel 120
Smith, J. P. 9
Snell-Rood, Claire 4, 120
social marginalization 92
social media 106
social organization and sensemaking 41
socio-cultural environment 19
Solimeo, Samantha 90
Sort and Sift, Think and Shift method 82–83, 85
Standards for Reporting Qualitative Research (SRQR) 108
Stange, K. C. 101
structured data collection tools, call sheet 47
surveys 9, 18–19, 34–35, 58, 98; background 81; broad brush 58; data 99; health 20
Swinglehurst, Deborah 59, 88

Tarrant, Carolyn 42
team-based ethnography 55–57; analyst(s) **56**; co-investigators **56**; project manager **56**; roles on an ethnographic team **56**; steps for conducting 55–57; team lead/principal investigator **56**
timeline maps 82
topic memos **78**, 80; *see also* memoing
traumatic brain injuries (TBIs) 64, 91
triangulation 8
True, Gala 47, 59, 64–66, 90–91, 121
trust 10, 43–44
Tuepker, Anaïs 59, 61–63

urban ethnography 79

video-reflexive ethnography 5, 58, 73, 106; observations 59
virtual ethnography 58
Visio software 9
visual displays 81, 104
Von Peter, Sebastian 121

Waller, Dylan 60–63
WhatsApp 119

Zatzick, Douglas 73
Zoom 58, 60